Problem Based Learning In Mental Retardation

Problem Based Learning In Mental Retardation

Dr. PS Reddy

Copyright © 2011 by Dr. PS Reddy.

ISBN: Softcover   978-1-4653-9726-3
           Ebook   978-1-4653-9727-0

All rights reserved. No part of this book may be reproduced or transmitted in any form or by any means, electronic or mechanical, including photocopying, recording, or by any information storage and retrieval system, without permission in writing from the copyright owner.

This book was printed in the United States of America.

To order additional copies of this book, contact:
Xlibris Corporation
0-800-644-6988
www.xlibrispublishing.co.uk
Orders@Xlibrispublishing.co.uk
303015

CONTENTS

Preface 9

1. Introduction 11
2. Terminology 21
3. Phenomenology 38
4. Comorbidity 52
5. Epidemiology 59
6. Aetiology of Mental Disorders 74
7. Psychiatric Assessment 86
8. Psychiatric Diagnosis 101
9. Psychiatric Syndromes 105
10. Psychopharmacology 117

Appendix 1 121
Appendix 2 129
Appendix 3 131
Appendix 4 133
Appendix 5 135
Appendix 6 137

References 139

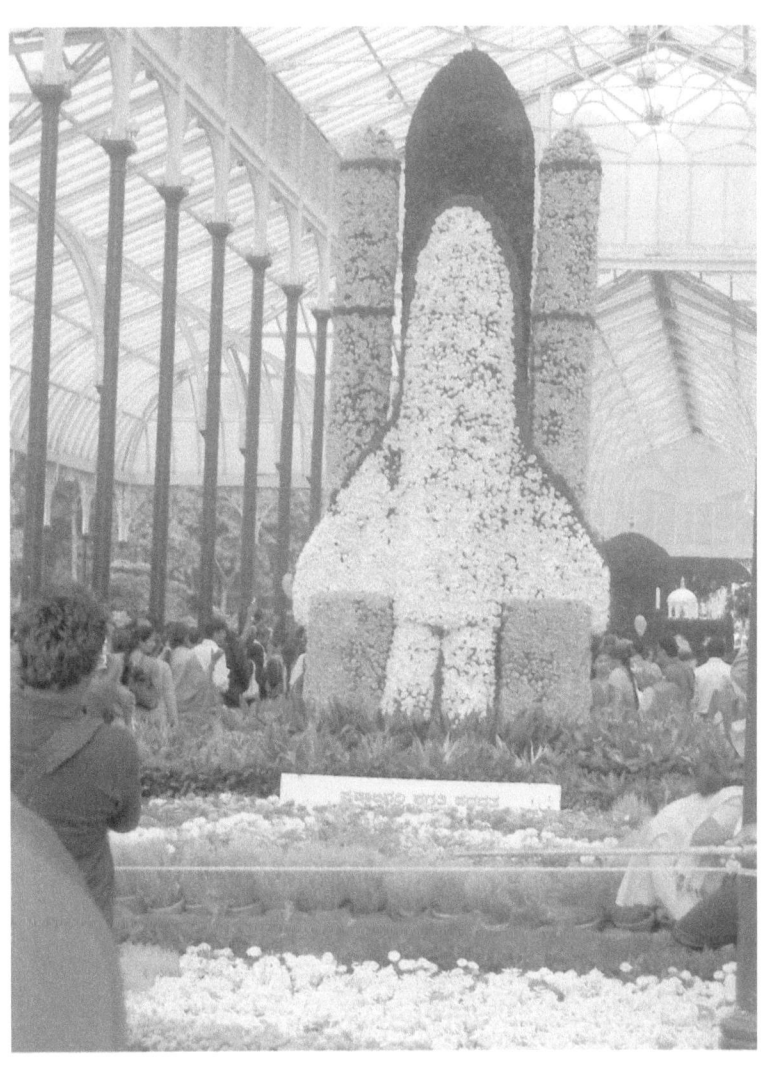

PREFACE

Problem based learning with a comprehensive assessment has been a positive step in evaluating trainees and students. This book attempts to provide a useful approach to understand learning disability and various concepts useful in assessment and management.

This book is not an indepth book but aims to aid in preparation for examinations.

The MCQ's are arranged in chapters to aid in understanding concepts and their relevance. The answers are provided nearby and other possible correct and wrong answers are mentioned to avoid duplicating MCQ's.

For more inquisitive readers additional material and references are presented. If you have any suggestions for improving the book please provide your constructive feedbacks to vidyarogya@gmail.com

Dr PS Reddy

INTRODUCTION

1. The term Mental Retardation is uncommonly used in routine clinical practice in the United Kingdom because

    1. The term Mental Retardation is unethical
    2. The term Mental Retardation is a recognized definition by the World Health Organisation
    3. The Royal college of Psychiatrists uses a different term
    4. The term Mental Retardation is socially inappropriate
    5. The term learning disability is preferred

    Answer: 5

    Learning disability is the common terminology used in the United Kingdom for mental retardation.

2. Current understanding of the concept of mental retardation in psychiatry does not include

    1. Etiological understanding of intelligence and its impairment,
    2. Assessment methods and management of for associated comorbidity
    3. Not clinically recognized as a developmental disorder
    4. Needs to meet criteria of impairment and dysfunction to be called disorder
    5. Intellectual impairment is essential for diagnosis of mental retardation

    Answer: 3

Correct Answers

- Clinically not identified as a developmental disorder
- Intellectual impairment alone is enough for diagnosis of mental retardation

Wong Answers

- Etiological understanding of intelligence and its impairment,
- Assessment methods and management of comorbid mental health disorders
- Identified clinically as a developmental disorder
- Needs to meet criteria of impairment and dysfunction to be called disorder

3. Various biopsychosociological factors are capable of producing deficits in intellectual function. These include

   1. Attention deficit hyperactivity disorder
   2. Autism
   3. Deprived sensory environment
   4. Sensory abnormalities
   5. All of the above

Answer: 5

Correct answers

- Attention deficit hyperactivity disorder
- Autism
- Deprived sensory environment
- Sensory abnormalities

Wrong answers

- Any potential cause after the age of 18 years

4. The co-occurrence of psychiatric illness with mental retardation

    1. Has not been well established
    2. People with mental retardation are more unlikely to suffer from mental disorders
    3. The change in prevalence of neuropsychiatric disorders is non specific
    4. Only prevalence of behavioural disorders, personality disorders, autistic spectrum disorders and attention—deficit hyperactivity disorder is affected.
    5. Has specific associated psychiatric syndromes associated as symptoms

Answer: 3

Correct Answers

- Has been well established
- People with learning disability are more unlikely to suffer from mental disorders
- The change in prevalence of neuropsychiatric disorders is non specific

Wrong Answers

- Has not been well established
- People with learning disability are more unlikely to suffer from mental disorders
- The change in prevalence of neuropsychiatric disorders is specific
- Only prevalence of behavioural disorders, personality disorders, autistic spectrum disorders and attention—deficit hyperactivity disorder is affected.
- Has specific associated psychiatric syndromes associated as symptoms

5. In people with learning disability, psychiatric disorders

    1. Are often overdiagnosed

2. Diagnostic overshadowing completely explains the difference in prevalence
3. Diagnostic overshadowing is not due to bias of clinicians
4. Diagnostic overshadowing is deliberate
5. Are often underdiagnosed

Answer: 5

Correct answers

- Are often underdiagnosed
- Diagnostic overshadowing does not completely explain the difference in prevalence
- Diagnostic overshadowing is due to bias of clinicians giving more emphasis to learning disability
- Diagnostic overshadowing is not deliberate

Wrong answers

- Are often overdiagnosed
- Diagnostic overshadowing completely explains the difference in prevalence
- Diagnostic overshadowing is not due to bias of clinicians
- Diagnostic overshadowing is deliberate

6. Masking in people with learning disability refers to

   1. Unemotional facial expression
   2. Presence of Autistic symptoms in severe learning disability
   3. Clinical characteristics of a mental disorder masked by a cognitive, language or speech deficit.
   4. People with learning disability share many mental health needs with the general population.
   5. Normalisation

   Answer: 3

Correct answers

- Clinical characteristics of a mental disorder masked by a cognitive, language or speech deficit

Wrong answers

- Unemotional facial expression
- Presence of Autistic symptoms in severe learning disability
- People with learning disability share many mental health needs with the general population.
- Normalisation

Diagnostic overshadowing is the tendency by which clinicians tend to overlook additional psychiatric diagnosis once a diagnosis of mental retardation is made. It is an observation bias.

Masking in phenomenology of learning disability refers to the clinical characteristics of a mental disorder being masked by a cognitive, language or speech deficits.

People with learning disability share many mental health needs with the general population but with increased prevalence. The increase in prevalence of neuropsychiatric disorders is generally considered to be non specific.

7. The earliest records of Mental retardation is from

   1. Vedas
   2. Old testament
   3. Papyri of Thebes
   4. New Testament
   5. Rome

Answer: 3

Correct answers

- Papyri of Thebes from Egypt (1500 B.C) Vedas

Wrong answers

- Old testament
- New Testament
- Rome

8. With regard to a famous book 'An Essay Concerning Human Understanding'

1. Written in 1689 by John Locke
2. Described that an individual is born with innate ideas
3. Described newborn mind as having inherent capabilities
4. Did not influence understanding of care and training provided to individuals with mental retardation.
5. Did not distinguish between mental retardation and mental illness.

Answer: 1

Correct answers

- Written in 1689 by John Locke
- Described that an individual is born without innate ideas
- Described mind as a 'tabula rasa', a blank slate.
- Profoundly influenced the understanding of care and training provided to individuals with learning disability
- Was the first book to distinguish between learning disability and mental illness.

Wrong answers

- The mind is born with inbuilt age activated capabilities
- Is the basis of biological understanding of inborn characters
- Explains temperament

Development of services and treatment of children with learning disability was the work done by a very dedicated physician Jean-Marc-Gaspard Itard. He worked in the National Institutes for Deaf Mutes in France to work with a boy named Victor who had apparently lived his whole life in the woods. He developed a training programme based on the work of John Locke who described the newborn brain as a clean slate 'Tabula Rosa' and Condillac who emphasized the importance of learning through the senses probably as a way of improving working memory. Itard used a broad educational program for Victor to develop his senses, intellectual functioning, attachment and emotions. After 5 years of training, Victor continued to have significant difficulties in language and social interaction. However he learned more skills and knowledge than many of his colleagues believed possible. Itard's educational approach including a humanistic attitude became widely accepted. It is even to this day used in the education of the deaf.

Itard later supervised Edouard Seguin who developed a comprehensive approach to the education of children with mental retardation, known as the Physiological Method. It included sensory training. Seguin moved to the United States where his ideas were given enough resources and backing. In 1876, he founded what would become the American Association of Metal Retardation.

9. The first test of intelligence

    1. Was developed by Binet
    2. Was developed by Henry Goddard
    3. Was introduced by Edgar Doll
    4. Was introduced by Kamat
    5. Was developed in America

Answer: 1

Correct answers

- Was developed by Binet
- Intelligence tests complement adaptive behaviour measurements

Wrong answers

- Was developed in America
- Was developed in the United Kingdom

- Is the Adult Intelligence Test
- Is the WAIS
- Is the WISC
- Adaptive behaviour cannot be measured and needs to be assessed by observation only
- Adaptive behaviour deficits are measured with intelligence tests

Binet's test of Intelligence was translated into English in 1908 by Henry Goddard. He later published an American version of the test. In 1935, Edgar Doll developed the Vineland Social Maturity Scale to assess the daily living skills/adaptive behavior of individuals suspected of having mental retardation.

Psychologists and educators now stepped in with medical professionals in believing that it was possible to determine who had mental retardation and provide appropriate training. Training schools later became centres breeding institutionalism. In the 1970's, a class action suit in Alabama established the right to treatment of individuals living in residential facilities. This legislation made purely custodial care no longer acceptable. The implications therefore include management of mental illness coexisting with mental retardation.

10. Performance subtests of WAIS-[R] include

1. Arithmetic
2. Object assembly
3. Picture completion
4. All the above
5. None of the above

Answer: 4

Correct answers

- Arithmetic
- Object assembly
- Picture completion

Wrong answers

- None of the above

11. 95% people have IQ of between

    1. 70 and 130
    2. 50 and 150
    3. 30 and 170
    4. 10 and 190
    5. 0 and 200

    Answer: 1

12. Verbal IQ in WAIS peaks

    1. Before the age of 10 years
    2. Before the age of 20 years
    3. Before the age of 30 years
    4. Before the age of 40 years
    5. Before the age of 50 years

    Answer: 5

TERMINOLOGY

1. Traditional terms denoting mental deficiency

    1. Do not predate psychiatric classification
    2. In North America the broad term 'developmental delay' has become an increasingly preferred synonym by parents and caregivers and is followed by professionals too
    3. In the UK the WHO terminology is used in routine clinical practice
    4. The term developmental disability is appropriate
    5. Intellectual disability and learning disability are increasingly being used as a synonym for people with significantly below-average intelligence

    Answer: 5

    Correct answers

    - Predate psychiatric classification
    - In North America the broad term 'developmental delay' has become an increasingly preferred synonym by parents and caregivers and is not followed by professionals too
    - In the UK the WHO terminology is not used in routine clinical practice
    - The term developmental disability is inappropriate and overinclusive
    - Intellectual disability and learning disability are increasingly being used as a synonym for people with significantly below-average intelligence

Wrong Answers

- Do not predate psychiatric classification
- In North America the broad term 'developmental delay' is not an increasingly preferred synonym by parents and caregivers
- In the UK the WHO terminology is used in routine clinical practice
- The term developmental disability is appropriate

Developmental disbility is a broad term including mental retardation and also to any other physical or psychiatric abnormality, such as delayed puberty.

Developmental delay has become an increasingly preferred synonym by parents and caregivers and is not followed by professionals because it is not a specific term.

2. Mental handicap is the term used by the

   1. UK Mental Health Act 1983
   2. Royal college of psychiatrists
   3. Department of Health
   4. Social Services
   5. Schools

Answer: 1

Correct answers

- UK Mental Health Act 1983 Royal college of psychiatrists

Wrong Answers

- Department of Health
- Social Services
- Schools

3. The term Mental Retardation is used by

   1. Oxford Textbook of Psychiatry
   2. American Association on Mental Retardation
   3. Diagnostic and Statistical Manual IV-DSM IV
   4. ICD-10
   5. All the above

   Answer: 5

   Correct Answers

   - Oxford Textbook of Psychiatry
   - American Association on Mental Retardation
   - Diagnostic and Statistical Manual IV-DSM IV
   - ICD-10
   - All the above

   Wrong Answers

   - Mental illness in Learning disability classification of the Royal college of psychiatrists in the United Kingdom

   Due to concern about the over identification or misidentification of mental retardation, particularly in minority populations and ethnic populations, the definition was revised to include an upper limit of IQ between 70-75 to account for IQ measurement error.

   The IQ performances resulting in scores of 71 through 75 are only consistent with mental retardation when significant deficits in adaptive behavior were present. However ICD and DSM do not consider this.

4. With regard to mental illness among people with learning disability

   1. Kraeplin described 'Pfropfschizophrenie'

2. Oligophrenia refers to mild learning disability with low psychic or mental functioning with psychopathology.
3. The types of psychopathology evident in patients with mental retardation
   Do not resemble those of normal individuals
4. Psychiatric disorders occur at normal frequency
5. All the above

Answer: 1

Correct answers

- Kraepelin described 'Pfropfschizophrenie'
- Oligophrenia refers to mild learning disability with low psychic or mental functioning without psychopathology.
- The types of psychopathology evident in patients with mental retardation resemble those of normal individuals
- Psychiatric disorders occur at a greater than normal frequency compared to general population

Wrong Answers

- Oligophrenia refers to mild learning disability with low psychic or mental functioning with psychopathology.
- The types of psychopathology evident in patients with mental retardation do not resemble those of normal individuals
- Psychiatric disorders occur at normal frequency

Epidemiological studies shows a greater than normal incidence of psychiatric disorders among children with learning disability. However specific mental disorders being necessarily associated with specific etiological forms of mental retardation is not conclusive.

Pfropfschizophrenie refers to schizophrenia overlapping on preexisting learning disability. Kraeplin also differentiated it from "oligophrenia", which refers to low psychic or mental functioning without presence of psychopathology seen in people with mild retardation, suggesting a neurodevelopmental origin.

5. An IQ measurement meeting ICD criteria for mental retardation

    1. Validates a disorder.
    2. Vast majority of people with mental retardation need no involvement from health and social services
    3. When otherwise healthy persons with mental retardation seek medical help their IQ needs to be assessed
    4. Their response is not influenced by temperament
    5. Inpatient treatment may be beneficial in general

Answer: 2

Correct answers

- Validates a disorder if adjustment restrictions are demonstrable.
- A vast majority of children and adults with mental retardation live in the community with very little need of involvement from health and social services and can be considered normal.
- Validates a disorder.
- When otherwise healthy persons with mental retardation seek medical help their IQ needs to be assessed
- Their response is not influenced by temperament
- Inpatient treatment may be beneficial in general

Wrong Answers

- When otherwise healthy persons with mental retardation seek medical help their IQ assessment is not always necessary
- Their response is influenced by temperament
- Inpatient treatment is not allways beneficial in general

6. In examining a person with learning disability for a physical problem

    1. Visiting a outpatient clinic may be less of an ordeal for the patient than admission.

2. Domiciliary visit in the presence of a carer is not ideal
3. Familiarity, dignity or independence do not mean much.
4. Elements of personal distress may mask or distort the objective signs and symptoms
5. Behaviour problems do not worsen when they are admitted as inpatients.

Answer: 4

Correct answers

- Visiting a outpatient clinic may be less of an ordeal for the patient than admission.
- Domiciliary visit in the presence of a carer is ideal
- Elements of personal distress may mask or distort the objective signs and symptoms
- Behaviour problems may worsen when they are admitted as inpatients

Wrong answers

- Visiting a outpatient clinic may be more of an ordeal for the patient than admission.
- Domiciliary visit in the presence of a carer is not ideal
- Familiarity, dignity or independence do not mean much
- Behaviour problems do not worsen when they are admitted as inpatients

7. Careful observations may need

1. Time to observe
2. Information from carers in interpreting symptoms.
3. A behavioural assessment and analysis to make sense
4. A detailed physical examination
5. All of the above

Answer: 5

Correct answers

- Time to observe
- Information from carers in interpreting symptoms.
- A behavioural assessment and analysis to make sense
- Detailed physical examination

Wrong Answers

- limited observation
- Information only from patient in interpreting symptoms.
- A psychoanalytic assessment and analysis to manage Learning Disability
- A detailed physical examination is not necessary

8. The American Association of Mental Retardation decided by consensus in 1993 that

   1. The term learning disability was most appropriate term
   2. The disability is characterized by significant limitations in intellectual functioning only
   3. The disability is characterized by significant limitations in adaptive behavior only
   4. This disability originates before the age of 18 years
   5. It is not used internationally

Answer: 4

Correct answers

- The term learning disability is non specific The disability is not characterized by significant limitations in intellectual functioning only
- The disability is not characterized by significant limitations in adaptive behavior only
- This disability originates before the age of 18 years
- It is used internationally

- The definition of mental retardation is concordant with the definition of the multidimensional International Classification of Impairments, Disabilities, and Handicaps from the World Health Organisation

Wrong Answers

- The term learning disability is the most appropriate term
- The disability is characterized by significant limitations in intellectual functioning only
- The disability is characterized by significant limitations in adaptive behavior only
- This disability originates after the age of 18 years
- It is not used internationally

Mental Retardation is the appropriate term. The disability is characterized by significant limitations both in intellectual functioning and in adaptive behavior as expressed in conceptual, social, and practical adaptive skills. Disability originates before the age of 18 years.

9. ICD 10 describes Mental Retardation as

   1. Arrested or incomplete development of the brain only 16 MCQs
   2. Impaired skills not manifested during developmental period
   3. Occuring always with mental or physical disorder
   4. Adaptive behaviour is not always impaired
   5. Vulnerable group for abuse and exploitation

Answer: 5

ICD-10 definition of mental retardation is arrested or incomplete development of the mind with Impaired skills manifesting as poor psychosocial adjustment. Impaired skills are manifested during developmental period. Can occur with or without mental or physical disorder. Adaptive behaviour is always impaired.

10. In assessing an individual with mental retardation a clinician should recognise

    1. Good functioning in a protected environment excludes mental retardation
    2. Assessment should not include culture and language
    3. Limitations excluding strengths
    4. With appropriate management perrson with mental retardation generally will improve
    5. All the above

Answer: 4

Correct answers

- Limitations in present functioning within the context of community environments typical of the individual's age peers and culture should be looked for and not just be content with good functioning in a protected enviornment.
- Assessment should include culture and language, differences in communication, sensory, motor, and behavioral factors.
- As with all normal people individuals limitations often coexist with strengths.
- With appropriate individualised support over a sustained period, the life functioning and adjustment of the person with mental retardation generally will improve.

Wrong Answers

- Good functioning in a protected enviornment.
- Assessment should not include culture and language
- Assessment should not include differences in communication, sensory, motor, and behavioral factors.
- Limitations do not coexist with strengths.
- With appropriate individualised support over a sustained period, the life functioning and adjustment of the person with mental retardation generally will become normal

11. With regard to intelligence

    1. It is a unitary concept
    2. Assessed on the basis of non specific skills
    3. Discrepencies in development of different skills developmentally is unusual Learning Disability: MCQs 17
    4. Discrepencies in development of different skills developmentally is abnormal
    5. All the above

    Answer: 3

    Correct answers

    - Discrepencies in development of different skills developmentally is unusual but is recognised

    Wrong Answers

    - It is a unitary concept
    - Assessed on the basis of non specific skills
    - Discrepencies in development of different skills developmentally is usual
    - Discrepencies in development of different skills developmentally is abnormal

12. The assessment of diagnostic category in which a person with mental retardation should be classified should be based on

    1. Clinical findings alone
    2. Adaptive behaviour judged in relation to individuals sociocultural background.
    3. ICD 10 or DSM IV Criteria
    4. Royal College Criteria
    5. Patient choice

    Answer: 3

Correct answers

- ICD 10 and DSM IV are generally accepted criteria

Wrong Answers

- Individual criteria are enough to make a diagnosis

13. Learning Disability

    1. Is a state which can vary
    2. Is a stable trait.
    3. Functioning is impaired
    4. May improve with appropriate input
    5. 1, 3 and 4

    Answer: 5

    Correct answers

    - Is a state which can vary
    - Functioning is impaired
    - May improve with appropriate input

    Wrong answers

    - Is a stable trait.
    - Functioning need not be impaired
    - Does not improve with appropriate input

14. Diagnostic and Statistical Manual of Mental Disorders—DSM IV definition of mental Retardation

    1. Does not reflect American Association on Mental Retardation definition
    2. Does not use severity level classification
    3. The upper IQ (Intelligence quotient) limit is 70

4. Comprehensive cognitive and adaptive skill assessment is necessary to make the diagnosis
5. Diagnosis should not be made on the basis of an outpatient visit or developmental screening.
6. All the above

Answer: 6

Correct answers

- Is the American Association on Mental Retardation definition
- Uses severity level classification
- The upper IQ (Intelligence quotient) limit for diagnosis of mental retardation is 70
- Comprehensive cognitive and adaptive skill assessment is necessary to make the diagnosis
- Diagnosis should not be made on the basis of an outpatient visit or developmental screening alone.

Wrong answers

- Is the ICD 9 definition
- Uses severity level classification
- The upper IQ for diagnosis of mental retardation is 100
- Comprehensive cognitive and adaptive skill assessment is not necessary to make the diagnosis
- Diagnosis should be made on the basis of an outpatient visit or developmental screening.

15. ICD 10 defines mental retardation as

1. A condition resulting only from a failure of the mind to develop completely
2. A condition resulting only from a arrest of the mind to develop
3. Like DSM-IV, ICD-10 suggests that cognitive, language; motor, social, and other adaptive behavior skills should all be used to determine the level of intellectual impairment

4. Does not support the idea of dual diagnosis
5. Four levels of mental retardation are specified in ICD-10: mild (IQ 50-69), moderate (IQ 35-49), severe (IQ 20-34), and profound (IQ below 20)

Answer: 5

Correct answers

- Four levels of mental retardation are specified in ICD-10: mild (IQ 50-69), moderate (IQ 35-49), severe (IQ 20-34), and profound (IQ below 20)
- A condition resulting only from a failure of the mind to develop completely

Wrong answers

- A condition resulting only from a arrest of the mind to develop Learning Disability
- ICD-10 suggests that cognitive, language; motor, social, and other adaptive behavior skills should all be used to determine the level of intellectual impairment in addition to IQ assessment
- Supports the idea of dual diagnosis
- Like DSM-IV, ICD-10 suggests that cognitive, language; motor, social, and other adaptive behavior skills should all be used to determine the level of intellectual impairment
- Does not support the idea of dual diagnosis
- Four levels of mental retardation are specified in ICD-10: mild (IQ 60-69), moderate (IQ 35-59), severe (IQ 20-34), and profound (IQ below 20)

16. People with mild mental retardation usually

1. Do not develop speech
2. Cannot engage in clinical interview
3. Cannot achieve full independence

4. Main difficulties are with regard to academic school work
   5. Cannot be helped in education

Answer: 4

Correct answers

- Develop speech
- Can engage in clinical interview
- Can achieve full independence
- Main difficulties are with regard to academic school work
- Can be helped in education

Wrong answers

- Do not develop speech
- Cannot engage in clinical interview
- Cannot achieve full independence
- Main difficulties are not with regard to academic school work
- Cannot be helped in education

17. People with moderate mental retardation usually have

   1. Limited language and comprehension skills
   2. Self care and motor skills are good
   3. They cannot learn the basic skills of reading, writing or counting
   4. As adults cannot do simple structured practical work
   5. Completely independent living is usual in adulthood

Answer: 1

Correct answers

- Limited language and comprehension skills
- Self care and motor skills need supervision
- They can learn the basic skills of reading, writing or counting

- As adults can do simple structured practical work
- Completely independent living is unusual in moderate learning disability adults

Wrong answers

- Good language and comprehension skills
- Self care and motor skills are good
- They cannot learn the basic skills of reading, writing or counting
- As adults cannot do simple structured practical work
- Completely independent living is usual in adulthood

18. In People with severe mental retardation

   1. The cause is unlikely to be of organic etiology
   2. Often do not have motor impairment or other neuropsychiatric sequelae
   3. Have good academic achievement
   4. Clinical picture is similar to moderate mental retardation
   5. All of the above

Answer: 4

Correct answers

- The cause is relatively likely to be of organic etiology
- Often have motor impairment or other neuropsychiatric sequelae
- Have poor academic achievement
- Clinical picture is similar to moderate mental retardation with associated neurological complications

Wrong answers

- The cause is relatively unlikely to be of organic etiology
- Often do not have motor impairment or other neuropsychiatric sequelae

- Have good academic achievement
- Clinical picture is not similar to moderate mental retardation

19. In people with profound mental retardation

   1. IQ is above 20
   2. Will not have basic understanding of commands and make simple requests
   3. Organic etiology cannot be identified in most people
   4. Neurological and physical disabilities are uncommon
   5. Psychiatric assessment of mental state can be possible

Answer: 5

Correct answers

- Psychiatric assessment of mental state can be possible with observation and interpretation with help from carer
- IQ is below 20

20. Marked clumsiness is commonly seen in

   1. Children with Asperger's Syndrome
   2. Children with Autism
   3. Children with mild learning disability
   4. All of the above
   5. None of the above

Answer: 2

Correct answers

- Not characteristic of Asperger's Syndrome
- Children with learning disability associated with neurological problems like cerebral palsy

Wrong answers

- Children with Asperger's Syndrome
- Children with learning disability

PHENOMENOLOGY

1. Psychopathology in mental retardation

   1. Can vary depending on the cognitive and intellectual ability
   2. Can vary depending on the level of communication
   3. Neurological and genetic phenotypes of mental retardation may present with unique symptoms.
   4. Observation and information from carer is an important diagnostic necessity
   5. All the above

   Answer: 5

   Correct answers

   - The description of symptoms can variable depending on the cognitive and intellectual ability
   - Can vary depending on the level of communication
   - Neurological and genetic phenotypes of mental retardation may present with unique symptoms.
   - Observation and information from carer is an important diagnostic necessity

   Wrong answers

   - Does not change depending on the cognitive and intellectual ability
   - Neurological and genetic phenotypes of mental retardation allways present with non specific symptoms.

- Observation and information from carer is not useful in diagnosis

2. Psychopathology associated with mental retardation can be discussed as:

   1. Developmental psychopathology of mental retardation
   2. Psychopathology of co morbid conditions of neurological and genetic origin
   3. Psychopathology of co morbid psychiatric disorders/mental illness
   4. All of the above
   5. None of the above

   Answer: 4

   Correct answers

   - Developmental psychopathology of mental retardation
   - Psychopathology of co morbid conditions of neurological and genetic origin
   - Psychopathology of co morbid psychiatric disorders/mental illness
   - Developmental psychopathology of mental retardation only
   - Psychopathology of co morbid conditions of neurological and genetic origin only
   - Psychopathology of co morbid psychiatric disorders/mental illness only

3. In people with Learning Disability having mental illness

   1. Psychiatric disorders are part of the learning disability
   2. Learning disability can contribute to the etiology of psychiatric and physical disorders
   3. Have a unique psychopathology of co morbid psychiatric disorders
   4. Diagnosis can sometimes be based on observation
   5. Do not have unique psychiatric syndromes associated with specific causes of learning disability

Answer: 5

Correct answers

- Psychiatric disorders are not always part of the learning disability and are usually mutually exclusive
- Learning disability can contribute to the etiology of psychiatric and physical disorders
- Have no uniqueness about psychopathology of specific co morbid psychiatric disorders
- Diagnosis can sometimes be based on observation
- Do not have unique psychiatric syndromes associated with specific causes of learning disability

Wrong answers

- Psychiatric disorders are part of the learning disability
- Learning disability does not contribute or is protective to the etiology of psychiatric and physical disorders
- Have a unique psychopathology of co morbid psychiatric disorders
- Diagnosis can sometimes be based on observation
- Have unique psychiatric syndromes associated with specific causes of learning disability

4. In a significant proportion

   1. Subtle signs of early developmental delay are allways noticed by parents and professionals
   2. Evidence of learning difficulties only become apparent at school
   3. Detailed assessment in learning disability is not essential to determine the types of effective interventions
   4. Systems of classification provide a useful framework for assessment
   5. All the above

Answer: 4

Correct answers

- Subtle signs of early developmental delay are allways noticed by parents and professionals
- Evidence of learning difficulties may only become apparent at school
- Detailed assessment of learning disability is essentially to determine need and to inform the types of effective intervention
- Systems of classification provide a useful framework for assessment
- Subtle signs of early developmental delay may remain unnoticed by parents and professionals
- Evidence of learning difficulties only become apparent at school
- Systems of classification do not provide a useful framework for assessment

5. People with Learning disability

   1. Cannot have severe impairments in one particular area
   2. Cannot have a particular area of higher skill.
   3. Can have severe impairments in one area and particular areas of higher skill
   4. All the above
   5. None of the above

Answer: 3

Correct answers

- Can have severe impairments in one area and particular areas of higher skill

For a definite diagnosis of learning disability, there should be a reduced level of intellectual functioning resulting in impairment in adaptive skills particularly in relation to normal social environment

6. DSM-IV diagnosis for Learning disability provides

    1. No framework for multiaxial diagnosis
    2. Axis III is for personality disorders and the level of mental retardation.
    3. Diagnosis of learning disability depends primarily on aetiology
    4. Focus is on quantifying the level of mental retardation.
    5. All the above

    Answer: 4

    Correct answers

    - Framework for multiaxial diagnosis
    - Axis II is for personality disorders and the level of mental retardation.
    - Diagnosis is not primarily one of aetiology Focus is on quantifying the level of mental retardation

    Wrong answers

    - No framework for multiaxial diagnosis Axis III is for personality disorders and the level of mental retardation.
    - Diagnosis of learning disability depends primarily on aetiology

7. Adaptive functions in learning disability

    1. Impaired depending on the level of intellectual functioning
    2. Used to determine the level of mental retardation
    3. Adaptive functioning has to be measured against what would be expected for a person of that age, and socio cultural background.
    4. All of the above
    5. None of the above

Answer: 4

Correct answers

- Impairment usually correlates with intellectual functioning
- Used to determine the level of mental retardation
- Adaptive functioning has to be measured

Wrong answers

- Impairment does not correlate with intellectual functioning
- Not useful to determine the level of mental retardation
- Adaptive functioning need not be measured against what would be expected for a person of that age, and socio cultural background against what would be expected for a person of that age, and socio cultural background

8. With regard to assessment of learning disability

   1. The Wechsler Intelligence Scale for adults is a validated instrument
   2. The Wechsler Intelligence Scale for adults is not a validated instrument
   3. Vineland Adaptive Behaviour Scales is a validated instrument
   4. Validation of a scale does not need normative data for comparison.
   5. Standardised procedures for diagnosis is not essential for accurate diagnosis of learning disability

Answer: 3

Correct answers

- The Wechsler Intelligence Scale for adults is a validated and reliable instrument
- Vineland Adaptive Behaviour Scales is a validated and reliable instrument
- Validation of a scale needs normative data for comparison.
- Standardised procedures for diagnosis is not essential for accurate diagnosis of learning disability

Wrong answers

- The Wechsler Intelligence Scale for adults is not a validated instrument
- Vineland Adaptive Behaviour Scales is not a validated instrument
- Validation of a scale does not need normative data for comparison.
- Standardised procedures for diagnosis is not essential for accurate diagnosis of learning disability

9. The diagnostic categories within mental retardation

   1. Are arbitrary divisions of a complex continuum.
   2. The diagnostic guidelines for mild, moderate, severe and profound mental retardation do not generally correspond to appropriate standardised IQ rating
   3. Are evidence based divisions of a simple continuum
   4. Are evidence based divisions of a complex continuum
   5. Are arbitrary divisions of a simple continuum

   Answer: 1

   Correct answers

   - Are arbitrary divisions of a complex continuum.
   - The diagnostic guidelines for mild, moderate, severe and profound mental retardation generally correspond to appropriate standardised IQ rating

   Wrong answers

   - The diagnostic guidelines for mild, moderate, severe and profound mental retardation do not generally correspond to appropriate standardised IQ rating
   - Are evidence based divisions of a simple continuum
   - Are not evidence based divisions of a simple continuum
   - Are not evidence based divisions of a complex continuum

- Are not arbitrary divisions of a simple continuum
- Are evidence based divisions of a complex continuum
- Are arbitrary divisions of a simple continuum

10. Challenging behaviour in learning disability is a

   1. Term to describe explain any behavioural disturbance
   2. Could result from a change in a particular behaviour in terms of intensity, frequency and duration that need not pose risk
   3. The term is borrowed from The American Association of Mental Retardation
   4. Challenging behaviour does not restrict access and opportunities for normalised psychosocial functioning
   5. Challenging behaviour is a final common pathway for many causes.

Answer: 5

Correct answers

- Challenging behaviour is a final common pathway for many causes
- It is a diagnosis by exclusion
- It is a clinical diagnosis

Wrong answers

- Term to describe explain any behavioural disturbance
- Could result from a change in a particular behaviour in terms of intensity, frequency and duration that need not pose risk
- The term is borrowed from The American Association of Mental Retardation
- Challenging behaviour does not restrict access and opportunities for normalised psychosocial functioning

Challenging behaviour is a term used to describe unexplained behavioural disturbance in people with learning disability.

Behavioural abnormality could result from a change in intensity, frequency and duration of preexisting habits or new behaviours that may pose risk to patients and others. The term was borrowed from The Association for Persons with Severe Handicaps (TASH). Challenging behaviour may restrict access and opportunities and worsen impairments and handicap. Challenging behaviour is a final common pathway for many causes.

---

11. Challenging behaviours in learning disability

    1. Does not include aggression
    2. Includes self-injurious behaviour
    3. Includes non-injurious stereo-typed behaviours with no risk of harm
    4. In ICD 10 cannot be included with the diagnosis of mental retardation
    5. In ICD 10 Impairment of behaviour is substituted by Challenging behaviour

Answer: 2

Correct answers

- Includes aggression both verbal and physical
- Includes self-injurious behaviour
- Includes non-injurious stereo-typed behaviours with risk of harm
- In ICD 10 can be included with the diagnosis of mental retardation
- In ICD 10 Impairment of behaviour is independent of Challenging behaviour

Wrong answers

- Does not include aggression
- Includes non-injurious stereo-typed behaviours with no risk of harm
- In ICD 10 cannot be included with the diagnosis of mental retardation

- In ICD 10 Impairment of behaviour is substituted by Challenging behaviour

12. Diagnosis of Challenging behaviour is not compliant with the following

    1. Is achieved by excluding all other causes
    2. Can be because of difficulty in communicating their needs to others
    3. The best way for carers to deal with challenging behaviour is to not worry about cause of the behaviour
    4. Needs observation by carers for a behavioural analysis.
    5. Challenging behaviour responds to medication if psychosocial interventions are ineffective.

    Answer: 3

    Correct answers

    - The best way for carers to deal with challenging behaviour is to not worry about cause of the behaviour

    Wrong answers

    - Is achieved by excluding all other causes
    - Can be because of difficulty in communicating their needs to others
    - The best way for carers to deal with challenging behaviour is to help lookout for cause of the behaviour
    - It needs observation by carers for a behavioural analysis.
    - Challenging behaviour responds to medication if psychosocial interventions are ineffective

13. Prevalence of challenging behaviour in Learning disability can be influenced by

    1. Social definition of challenging behaviour
    2. Individual perception of carers
    3. Individual circumstances

4. May start in early childhood and do not continue into adulthood
5. 1, 2, 3

28 MCQs

Answer: 5

Correct answers

- Social definition of challenging behaviour
- Individual perception of carers
- Individual circumstances
- May start in early childhood and often continue into adulthood

Wrong answers

- May start in early childhood and do not continue into adulthood

14. Challenging behaviour is

1. Less common in men
2. Uncommon in those with comorbid autistic spectrum disorder
3. Uncommon if additional disabilities result in abnormal senory perception and communication
4. In the severely learning disabled
5. All the above

Answer: 4

Correct answers

- More common in men/boys
- More common in those with comorbid autistic spectrum disorder
- More common if additional disabilities result in abnormal sensory perception and communication
- In the severely learning disabled

Wrong answers

- Less common in men
- Uncommon in those with comorbid autistic spectrum disorder
- Uncommon if additional disabilities result in abnormal senory perception and communication
- In the less severely learning disabled

15. In managing Challenging behavior

   1. There is no need to exclude mental health problems such as depression
   2. Do not benefit from individually planned behavioural assessments
   3. Relaxation is unhelpful
   4. Social skills may not help people manage their anger or social anxiety.
   5. Cognitive-behavioural approaches are useful.

Answer: 5

Correct answers

- Psychiatric syndromes may present with atypical symptoms and need to be carefully evaluated

Wrong answers

- Do not benefit from individually planned behavioural assessments
- Relaxation is unhelpful
- Learning disability is not a contraindication for cognitive behaviour therapy
- Social skills may not help people manage their anger or social anxiety.
- Cognitive-behavioural approaches are unhelpful

16. Abnormalities of stream of thought

    1. Can be seen in poverty of thought
    2. Is a symptom of learning disability
    3. Is a sign of learning disability
    4. Is characteristic of learning disability
    5. Is pathognomonic of learning disability

Answer: 1.

Correct answers

- Can be seen in poverty of thought
- Can be a symptom of learning disability
- Can be a sign of learning disability
- Is not characteristic of learning disability
- Is not pathognomonic of learning disability

Wrong answers

- Is a symptom of learning disability
- Is a sign of learning disability
- Is characteristic of learning disability
- Is pathognomonic of learning disability

17. Obsessive compulsive symptoms are often usual symptoms of

    1. Mild learning disability
    2. Patients with severe depression
    3. Autism
    4. Rett's syndrome
    5. All of the above

Answer: 5

Correct answers

- Patients with severe depression

- Autism
- Rett's syndrome
- All of the above
- Severe learning disability

Wrong answers

- Mild learning disability

COMORBIDITY

1. Genetic disorders are

    1. Not associated with mental retardation
    2. Have no causal role in mental retardation
    3. Cannot be comorbid causes only
    4. Causal relationships must be inferred
    5. Can be classified as prenatal causes, perinatal causes, and postnatal causes

    Answer: 4

    Correct answers

    - Can be associated
    - Can have causal role
    - Causal relationships must be inferred

    Wrong Answer

    - Can be classified as prenatal causes, perinatal causes, and postnatal causes

2. Causes associated with mental retardation are classified into

    1. Prenatal causes
    2. Perinatal causes

3. Postnatal causes
4. All
5. None

Answer: 4

Correct answers

- Temporal association of cause can be classified into pre, peri and postnatal

3. The classification systems for mental retardation recognize

   1. The need to focus on capabilities
   2. The need to focus on disability
   3. The level of support required
   4. Learning disability can be a symptom of other disorders as well as a unique syndrome
   5. All of the above

Answer: 5

Correct answers

- Abilities and disabilities are important in assessment and later management

Wrong Answer

- Disabilities alone need to be evaluated

4. Among the factors associated with severe mental retardation

   1. Chromosomal abnormality is relatively uncommon
   2. Genetic causes are uncommon in individuals with severe mental retardation

3. Perinatal factors such as perinatal hypoxia and obstetric complications are increasing
4. Postnatal factors such as brain trauma are increasing
5. Down's Syndrome is a common genetic cause of learning disability

Answer: 5

Correct answers

- Chromosomal abnormality is more common factor associated with severe learning disability

Wrong Answer

- Perinatal factors such as perinatal hypoxia and obstetric complications are increasing

Genetic causes are more common in individuals with severe mental retardation

Perinatal factors and postnatal factors are decreasing causes

5. Neurological conditions associated with learning disability include

   1. Epilepsy
   2. Autism
   3. Increased risk of tardive dyskinesia to typical antipsychotics
   4. Abnormalities on detailed neurological assessment
   5. All the above

Answer: 5

Correct answers

- Epilepsy
- Autism

- Increased risk of tardive dyskinesia to typical antipsychotics
- Abnormalities on detailed neurological assessment

Wrong Answer

- No increased risk of nerological disorders
- No increased risk of physical disorders

6. In eliciting psychopathology among people with learning disability

   1. Expression of moods and feelings is reliable
   2. Clarity and structure of cognitive symptoms is not restricted
   3. There are universally agreed criteria for diagnosis
   4. Diagnosis may need to be based on behavioural observations and course of illness
   5. All the above

Answer 4

Correct answers

- Diagnosis may need to be based on behavioural observations and course of illness
- Criteria for diagnosis are generalized from ICD 10 and DSM IV and may not be appropriate in more severe forms of learning disability

Wrong Answer

- Expression of moods and feelings may not be communicated well
- Clarity and structure of cognitive symptoms is not restricted
- There are universally agreed criteria for diagnosis

7. Specific learning disability in reading is associated with

    1. Soft neurological signs
    2. Exaggerated deep tendon reflexes
    3. Bilateral plantar extensor responses
    4. All the above
    5. None of the above

    Answer: 1

    Correct answers

    - Soft neurological signs

    Wrong Answer

    - Exaggerated deep tendon reflexes
    - Bilateral plantar extensor responses

8. Female physical characteristics are present in the

    1. People with Klinefelter's syndrome
    2. Down's syndrome
    3. Turner's syndrome
    4. Males with Eating disorder
    5. None of the above

    Answer: 3

    Correct answers

    - People with Turner's syndrome

    Wrong Answer

    - People with Klinefelter's syndrome
    - Down's syndrome

- Turner's syndrome
- Males with Eating disorder

9. Very Intelligent people and patients are

    1. Less likely to respond to placebo
    2. More likely to respond to placebo
    3. Do not respond to placebo
    4. Do not have specific learning difficulties
    5. Do not have specific learning disabilities

Answer: 1

Correct answers

- Less likely to respond to placebo
- Can respond to placebo
- Can have specific learning difficulties
- Can have specific learning disabilities

Wrong Answer

- More likely to respond to placebo
- Do not respond to placebo
- Do not have specific learning difficulties
- Do not have specific learning disabilities

10. Specific reading difficulties are

    1. Significantly associated with males
    2. Significantly associated with females
    3. Early detection is unhelpful
    4. Can only be detected late in life
    5. Associated with gross neurological signs

Answer:

Correct answers

- Significantly associated with males
- Not significantly associated with females
- Early detection is helpful
- Can be managed by remedial education
- May be detected late in life
- May be unnoticed in primary school
- Associated with soft neurological signs

Wrong Answer

- Not significantly associated with males
- Significantly associated with females
- Early detection is unhelpful
- Can only be detected late in life
- Associated with gross neurological signs

EPIDEMIOLOGY

1. The reasons for difficulties in estimating prevalence of mental disorders in people with learning disability include

   1. Variable terminology
   2. Ill-defined syndromes
   3. Culture-specific and changeable social labels
   4. Stigma
   5. All the above

   Answer: 1

   Correct answers

   - Variable terminology
   - Categories of mental retardation are well defined
   - Difficulty in obtaining self report responses

   Wrong Answer

   - Ill-defined syndromes
   - Culture-specific and changeable social labels
   - Stigma

2. The general health of people with learning disability is

   1. Very poor in Down's syndrome compared to other causes
   2. Is better than that of the general population

3. Restricted to increased neuropsychiatric sequelae
4. Obesity and physical illnesses are also increased
5. All of the above

Answer: 4

Correct answers

- Obesity and physical illnesses are also increased.
- Increased neuropsychiatric sequelae

Wrong Answer

- Very poor in Down's syndrome compared to other causes
- Is better than that of the general population
- Restricted to increased neuropsychiatric sequelae

3. International differences in prevalence, quality of life, morbidity, and life expectancy for people with learning disability are

   1. Very similar
   2. The increase is in prevalence of severe retardation compared to milder forms
   3. The increase is due to increased incidence of Down's syndrome
   4. Economic deprivation accounts for all the difference
   5. Health, education and social services can make a difference

Answer: 5

Correct answers

- Very variable
- The increase is in prevalence of severe retardation compared to milder forms
- Economic deprivation does not account for all the difference
- The increased incidence of Down's syndrome has been noticed in cultures where age of conception has increased

Wrong Answer

- Very similar
- The increase is in prevalence of milder forms of mental retardation compared to severe mental retardation
- Economic deprivation accounts for all the difference

The World Health Organisation has defined ways of conceptualising deviation from normal health. These concepts include

Impairment: Loss or abnormality of psychological, physiological or physical structure or function

Disability: Reduction or inability of ability resulting from impairment

Handicap: Is a disadvantage resulting from disability that limits the fulfillment of ones potential

---

4. Prevalence varies between different communities with similar socio economic background.

   1. Similar births cohorts in different communities
   2. Greater variation is seen in developing countries
   3. Environmental factors like iodine deficiency disease can explain such variation
   4. Age-specific prevalence may vary over time in the same community
   5. All the above

Answer: 5

Correct answers

- Similar births cohorts in different communities
- Greater variation is seen in developing countries

- Environmental factors like iodine deficiency disease can explain such variation
- Age-specific prevalence may vary over time in the same community

Wrong Answer

- Variation is not seen in countries with same socioeconomic status
- Greater variation is seen in developed countries
- Enviornmental factors do not contribute to variations in prevalence

5. Among aetiologically recognized syndromes

   1. Down's syndrome is not a common group
   2. Down's syndrome may be more in communities where late conception is prevalent.
   3. Preventive programmes cannot identify Down's syndrome prenatally
   4. Preventive programmes can prevent Down's syndrome prior to conception
   5. Fragile X is an uncommon cause

Answer: 2

Correct answers

- Down's syndrome may be more in communities where late conception is prevalent.
- Preventive programmes can identify Down's syndrome prenatally

Wrong Answer

- Preventive programmes cannot identify Down's syndrome prenatally
- Preventive programmes can prevent Down's syndrome prior to conception

6. Factors reducing prevalence of learning disability

   1. Treating maternal inherited metabolic disorders and hypothyroidism
   2. Perinatal factors now produce more neurological impairments
   3. Immunization has not reduced teratogenic infectious diseases
   4. Early stimulation and training in management has improved function.
   5. All the above

   Answer: 4

   Correct answers

   - Early screening and treatment for inherited metabolic disorders and hypothyroidism
   - Perinatal factors produce fewer neurological impairments
   - Immunization has reduced teratogenic infectious diseases
   - Early stimulation and training in management has improved function

   Wrong Answer

   - Treating maternal inherited metabolic disorders and hypothyroidism
   - Perinatal factors now produce more neurological impairments
   - Immunization has not reduced teratogenic infectious diseases

7. Prevalence of learning disability may vary by age because

   1. Prenatal interventions may change over time
   2. Postnatal interventions may change over time
   3. Peri natal interventions change over time
   4. Survival has increased at all ages and this may affect prevalence of different causes of mental retardation.
   5. All the above

Answer: 5

8. With regard to prevalence of learning disability in the UK

    1. Prevalence data alone can be used to estimate age-specific prevalence ratios
    2. Mortality data alone can be used to estimate age-specific prevalence ratios
    3. There are usually more males than females at all ages
    4. Evidence suggests lack of a social class gradient
    5. Evidence suggesting lack of social class gradient may be because of confounding variables.

Answer: 3

Correct answers

- Evidence suggests lack of a social class gradient

Wrong Answer

- Prevalence data alone can be used to estimate age-specific prevalence ratios
- Mortality data alone can be used to estimate age-specific prevalence ratios
- There are usually more males than females at all ages

9. In children with mild intellectual impairment

    1. Many are identified only at school
    2. Minor delays in milestones are very sensitive in diagnosis
    3. Can communicate without difficulty
    4. All the above
    5. None of the above

Answer: 4

Correct answers

- Many are identified only at school
- Minor delays in milestones are very sensitive in diagnosis

Wrong Answer

- Gross nerological deficits are common

The term Borderline learning disability was USA and was removed because of recognized abuses perpetrated on people with such a non specific diagnosis. Many young women were institutionalized especially when pregnant and children adopted.

10. Children with mild learning disability are more likely to be labeled or identified if they also have

1. No history of epilepsy
2. No communication problems
3. No physical disabilities
4. Associated Mental illness or challenging behaviour
5. Low socio economic status

Answer: 4

Correct answers

- History of epilepsy
- Communication problems
- Associated Mental illness or challenging behaviour
- High socio economic status

Wrong Answer

- No communication problems
- No physical disabilities

- No associated mental illness or challenging behaviour
- Low socio economic status

11. Adults with mild learning disability are more likely to be labeled or identified if they also are

   1. Employed
   2. Low socio-economic status
   3. Poor home environment
   4. All of the above
   5. Exhibit inadequate parental care towards their children

   Answer: 5

   Correct answers

   - Exhibit inadequate parental care towards their children

   Wrong Answer

   - Employed
   - Low socio-economic status
   - Poor home environment

12. Prevalence of mild learning disability in developing countries
    Learning Disability: MCQs 39

    1. Variable differences are not related to the varying preventable causes
    2. The variability is more a marker of health, social and education than to do with economics alone
    3. Due to methodological difficulties mild mental retardation prevalence rates are more reliable
    4. Severe mental retardation prevalence rates are less reliable
    5. All the above

    Answer: 2

Correct answers

- Variable differences may be related to varying preventable causes
- The variability is more a marker of health, social and education along with economics
- Due to methodological difficulties mild mental retardation prevalence rates are less reliable
- Severe mental retardation prevalence rates are more reliable

Wrong Answer

- Variable differences are not related to the varying preventable causes
- Due to methodological difficulties mild mental retardation prevalence rates are more reliable
- Severe mental retardation prevalence rates are less reliable

13. For individuals with severe learning disability

1. The disabilities do not necessitate special supports and services
2. In epidemiological studies it has often been defined and identified according to the level of service need
3. Prevalence is considered to be a less reliable estimate of true prevalence
4. Severe intellectual impairment is often recognised late
5. None of the above

Answer: 2

Correct answers

- In epidemiological studies it has often been defined and identified according to the level of service need

Wrong Answer

- Disabilities do not necessitate special supports and services

- Prevalence is considered to be a less reliable estimate of true prevalence
- Severe intellectual impairment is often recognised late

The severe learning disability necessitates support services. In epidemiological studies severe learning disabilities is identified according to the level of service need. Severe learning disability prevalence is more reliable than milder forms. Severe intellectual impairment is recognised earlier. A comparative study in nine countries showed similar figures. Only in Southern India migration was considered a cause for high teenage figures of severe mental retardation.

14. Precise comparative statistics between countries

    1. Is important especially for mental retardation.
    2. It is not important to identify locally preventable etiological factors
    3. Local preventable factors cannot be strategically managed
    4. Local preventable factors should be managed for each individual patient
    5. None of the above

Answer: 5

Correct answers

- Local preventable factors can be strategically managed

Wrong Answer

- Local preventable factors cannot be strategically managed
- Local preventable factors should be managed for each individual patient

15. Eliciting psychopathology in learning disability needs to overcome

    1. Challenges of developmental psychopathology
    2. Easy communication by people with learning disability
    3. Unreliable symptoms of specific psychiatric disorders
    4. Lack of evidence from research
    5. All of the above

Answer: 1

Correct answers

- Challenge of developmental psychopathology
- Communication difficulties in people with learning disability
- Variable and atypical symptoms of specific psychiatric disorders
- There is some evidence from research

Wrong Answer

- Easy communication by people with learning disability
- Unreliable symptoms of specific psychiatric disorders
- Lack of evidence from research

Studies into the prevalence of psychiatric illness among adults with intellectual disability report a wide range, between 10%-39%.

16. Rate of psychiatric illness in learning disability increases with

    1. Severity of intellectual disability
    2. Schizophrenia and psychoses in particular are more prevalent in severe and profound learning disability
    3. Psychiatric morbidity increases with age

4. In adults aged 50 years and over rates of dementia is lower than normal population
5. None of the above

Answer: 2

Correct answers

- Schizophrenia and psychoses in particular are more prevalent in severe and profound learning disabilities
- In adults aged 50 years and over rates of dementia is higher than normal population

Wrong Answer

- Psychiatric morbidity increases with age
- In adults aged 50 years and over rates of dementia is lower than normal population except for Down's syndrome

17. With regard to people with learning disability

1. Rates of psychiatric illness with intellectual disabilities and epilepsy are significantly different from those with no epileptsy
2. Rates of behavioural disorder with intellectual disabilities and epilepsy are significantly different from those with no epileptsy
3. Rates of psychiatric illness with intellectual disabilities and epilepsy are not significantly different from those with no epileptsy
4. Rates of behavioural disorder in adults with intellectual disabilities and epilepsy are not significantly different from those with no epilepsy
5. Rates of behavioural disorder and psychiatric illness with intellectual disabilities and epilepsy are not significantly different from those with no epilepsy

Answer: 5

Correct answers

- Epilepsy is more commonly associated with learning disability

Wrong Answer

- Epilepsy does not affect prevalence of mental illness in those with learning disability

18. With regard to learning disability due to Down's syndrome

   1. Psychiatric disorders in adults with severe intellectual disabilities but not Down's syndrome is higher than in adults with intellectual disabilities and Down's syndrome
   2. The rate of depression is higher
   3. Dementia is less common
   4. Cardiac malformations are less common
   5. None the above

Answer: 5

19. Prevalence of specific psychiatric illnesses amongst adults with intellectual disability

   1. Indicate that some are more prevalent than others in people with intellectual disability
   2. The prevalence of schizophrenia is increased
   3. The prevalence of affective disorders including depressive illness and mania are decreased
   4. The point prevalence of anxiety related disorders in adults is decreased
   5. Prevalence of ADHD is lesser than in children with average intelligence

Answer: 2

Correct answers

- The prevalence of schizophrenia is increased
- Prevalence of ADHD is higher than in children with average intelligence

Wrong Answer

- The prevalence of ADHD amongst adults with severe and profound intellectual disability is not similar to children with severe intellectual disability

20. Among children and adults with learning disability

   1. Aggression is associated with 40% of depressed people
   2. Outreach treatment is ineffective alternative to hospital treatment
   3. Outreach treatment is inefficient alternative to hospital treatment
   4. Assertive community outreach treatment or intensive care can significantly increase hospital admission
   5. Referrals to psychiatrists as emergencies presented with behavioural problems less commonly

Answer: 1

Correct answers

- Aggression is associated with 40% of depressed people
- Agression may be a symptom of communication difficulties

Wrong Answer

- Outreach treatment is ineffective alternative to hospital treatment
- Outreach treatment is inefficient alternative to hospital treatment

- Assertive community outreach treatment or intensive care can significantly increase hospital admission
- Referrals to psychiatrists as emergencies presented with behavioural problems less commonly

AETIOLOGY OF MENTAL DISORDERS

1. Aetiological factors among people with learning disability

    1. Multifactorial causative factors are uncommon
    2. Historically biological causative factors were disregarded
    3. Psychosocial factors are primary to aetiology of mental disorders
    4. Uniqueness of phenotypic behavioural epiphenomena associated with genetic syndromes is diagnostic
    5. People with mental retardation need genetic testing for diagnosis

Answer 5

Correct answers

- Multifactorial causative factors contribute to aetiology of mental illness
- Historically biological causative factors took precedence
- Psychosocial factors play a secondary role in aetiology of mental disorders
- Uniqueness of phenotypic behavioural epiphenomena associated with genetic syndromes is not diagnostic
- People with mental retardation need genetic testing for confirming diagnosis

Wrong Answer

- Multifactorial causative factors are uncommon
- Historically biological causative factors were disregarded

- Psychosocial factors are primary to aetiology of mental disorders
- Uniqueness of phenotypic behavioural epiphenomena associated with genetic syndromes is diagnostic

2. In some genetic syndromes

   1. Characteristic behavioural symptoms may not aid in diagnosis
   2. Characteristic dysmorphic features may not aid in diagnosis
   3. Characteristic behavioural symptoms may aid in diagnosis
   4. Characteristic dysmorphic features may aid in diagnosis
   5. Characteristic behavioural symptoms and dysmorphic features may aid in diagnosis

Answer: 5

Correct answers

- Behaviour and clinical findings are suggestive in most patients
- Genetic testing is diagnostic

Wrong Answer

- Genetic testing is unnecessary to rule out common causes of mental retardation

Some pathognomonic signs are diagnostic. Common examples include Wilsons Disease and Tuberous sclerosis

3. In understanding behavioural phenotypes of learning disability

   1. The most widely studied is the Down's syndrome
   2. The association between Down's syndrome and psychiatric disorders is clear
   3. Improved understanding has mystified aetiology of challenging behaviour

4. Behavioural phenotype has helped in understanding aetiology of Down's syndrome
   5. None of the above

Answer: 1

Correct answers

- The most widely studied are Down's syndrome and Fragile X

Wrong Answer

- The association between Down's syndrome and psychiatric disorders is clear
- Improved understanding has mystified aetiology of challenging behaviour
- Behavioural phenotype has helped in understanding aetiology of Down's syndrome

4. With regard to behavioural disturbance and learning difficulties

   1. There is increasing evidence that behavioural disturbances are always related to psychiatric disorders
   2. A chain of constraining psychosocial and environmental events is allways set off by a single factor
   3. Understanding aetiology does not aid in management
   4. Psychosocial and environmental factors are the only therapeutically modifiable factors
   5. Psychosocial and environmental interventions have proven long term benefits

Answer: 5

Correct answers

- A chain of constraining psychosocial and environmental events can be set off by a single factor

Wrong Answer

- Understanding aetiology does not aid in management
- Psychosocial and environmental factors are the only therapeutically modifiable factors

5. In learning disability with challenging behaviours

   1. Can be difficult to establish cause
   2. Can be a presentation of adjustment problems, physical illness or psychiatric disorder
   3. Comprehensive aetiological formulation is not needed in planning intervention
   4. Behavioural disturbance augments the impairment of mental retardation resulting in increasing care needs
   5. All of the above

   Answer: 5

6. The association of mental disorder and learning disability could be

   1. Chance association of psychiatric disorder with mental retardation
   2. Increased incidence of psychiatric disorders among people with mental retardation
   3. Decreased incidence of psychiatric disorders among people with mental retardation
   4. 1 and 2
   5. None of the above

   Answer: 4

Correct answers

- Chance association of psychiatric disorder with mental retardation
- Increased incidence of psychiatric disorders among people with mental retardation

Wrong Answer

- Decreased incidence of psychiatric disorders among people with mental retardation

7. The problems in evaluating probable associations between learning disability and mental illness are

   1. Diagnostic undershadowing
   2. Understanding relevance of neurodevelopmental processes in aberrant behaviour
   3. Specificity of aetiological association
   4. Absence of comorbid neurodevelopment disorders
   5. Evidence for later/earlier onset of psychiatric illnesses

Answer: 2

Correct answers

- Diagnostic overshadowing
- Understanding relevance of neurodevelopmental processes in aberrant behaviour
- Lack of specificity of aetiological association Co morbid neurodevelopment disorders
- Lack of evidence for later/earlier onset of psychiatric illnesses
- Studies specifically studying association between mental retardation and psychiatric disorders are relatively few

Wrong Answers

- Diagnostic undershadowing
- Specificity of aetiological association
- Absence of comorbid neurodevelopment disorders
- Evidence for later/earlier onset of psychiatric illnesses

8. Among comobid psychiatric disorders in people with learning disability

    1. Improved diagnostic tools have not enabled more reliable research
    2. Affective disorder as the commonest psychiatric diagnosis
    3. The lifetime risk of schizophrenia is 3 times more than in general population
    4. Mania is rare compared to general population
    5. Autism is rare compared to general population

Answer: 2

Correct answers

- Improved diagnostic tools have enabled more reliable research
- Affective disorders are the commonest psychiatric diagnosis
- The lifetime risk of schizophrenia is more than in general population
- Autism is more common compared to general population

Wrong Answers

- Improved diagnostic tools have not enabled more reliable research
- Anxiety disorder is the commonest psychiatric diagnosis
- The lifetime risk of schizophrenia is 3 times more than in general population
- Mania is rare compared to general population

9. The needs of the individual with both learning disability and mental illness are

    1. Not overshadowed by a primary diagnosis of mental retardation
    2. Overshadowing involves an emphasis of treatment on learning disability rather than mental illness

3. Masking can explain the difference of management
4. Masking cannot explain the undiagnosed mental illness
5. Better managed one after the other

Answer: 2

10. Mental illnesses in learning disability

    1. Can be neurodevelopmental
       Learning Disability: MCQs 47
    2. Pathological insults and the temporal relationship between intrauterine injury and to early onset schizophrenia have been reported
    3. The extent of intrauterine injury change confounding the association between mental retardation and schizophrenia is clear
    4. Has a different aetiological cascade
    5. None of the above

Answer: 2

Correct answers

- Pathological insults and the temporal relationship between intrauterine injury and to early onset schizophrenia have been reported

Wrong Answers

- Can be neurodevelopmental
- Has a different aetiological cascade

11. With regard to mental illness and mental retardation

    1. No evidence to suggest neurodevelopmental factors in aetiology
    2. In very low birth weight babies pervasive developmental disorder are increased
    3. In very low birth weight babies attention-deficit hyperactivity disorders are not increased

4. There is no association between low birth weight, premature birth and learning disability
5. None of the above

Answer: 2

Correct answers

- In very low birth weight babies, functional disorders caused by subtle neurological damage such as attention-deficit hyperactivity disorders and pervasive developmental disorder are also increased

Wrong Answers

- There is no association between low birth weight, premature birth and learning disability

12. Among people with learning disability

1. Comorbid neurodevelopmental disorders often coexist
2. Pervasive developmental disorders are uncommon
3. Epilepsy is uncommon
4. Epilepsy and Pervasive developmental disorders are commonest comorbid neurodevelopmental disorders
5. 1 and 4

Answer: 5

Some toddlers with autism lose their skills at around 18 months although this may even happen in adolescence. This widely reported deterioration may possibly be a relatively small environmental insult destabilizing an immature or genetically predisposed brain. It is called developmental regression and has been documented as evidence based.

13. The age of onset of disorders in people with mental retardation

    1. Is not specific for most psychiatric disorders
    2. Congenital maformations are not noticeable at birth
    3. Adults with Down's syndrome and other adults with learning disability do not have increased risk of dementia
    4. Adults with Down's syndrome have increased risk of Alzheimer's dementia compared to others
    5. A few common genetic syndromes have a degenerative course associated with progressive cognitive deficits.

    Answer: 4

A few rare genetic syndromes have a degenerative course associated with progressive cognitive deficits.

---

14. Compared to prevalence of psychiatric disorders in normal population

    1. Mental illness prevalence among people with mental retardation is the same.
    2. Studies of psychiatric morbidity have no methodological problems
    3. Difficulties in ascertaining diagnosis by self rating is not a limiting factor in validity
    4. The disability resulting from psychiatric disorder and learning disability results in handicap and impairment resulting in more than just adding up individually resulting impairments
    5. The disability resulting from psychiatric disorder and learning disability results in impairment accounted by just adding up individually resulting impairments

    Answer: 4

    Correct answers

    - The disability resulting from psychiatric disorder and learning disability results in handicap and impairment resulting in more than just adding up individually resulting impairments

Wrong Answers

- Mental illness prevalence among people with mental retardation is the same.
- Studies of psychiatric morbidity have no methodological problems

15. The disability caused by learning disability results from

    1. Loss of social opportunities
    2. Loss of educational opportunities
       Learning Disability: MCQs 49
    3. Loss of psychological opportunities
    4. Loss of self esteem
    5. All of the above

    Answer: 5

16. The disability caused by institutionalism in people with learning disability can result in

    1. Lack of personal stress
    2. No distress for carers
    3. No long term increased cost to the community
    4. Are increasingly being minimized by closing large hospitals
    5. None of the above

    Answer: 4

    Correct answers

    - Causes personal stress, devalues people, promotes loosing skills for daily living and self help skills
    - Are increasingly being minimized by closing large hospitals

Wrong Answers

- Lack of personal stress
- No distress for carers

17. Studies in people with learning disability and mental disorder

    1. Have questioned the contributory risk of mental retardation to mental illness
    2. The aetiologic role of mental retardation can be as a vulnerability factor
    3. The stress vunerability hypothesis cannot apply to people with learning disability
    4. Syndromes have no well established association with behavioural difficulties and self harm
    5. None of the above

Answer: 2

Correct answers

- The aetiologic role of mental retardation can be as a vulnerability factor

Wrong Answers

- The stress vunerability hypothesis cannot apply to people with learning disability
- Syndromes have no well established association with behavioural difficulties and self harm

18. With regard to learning disability

    1. Lesch Nyhan syndrome is associated with self injurious behaviour
    2. Prader—Willi syndrome is not associated with obesity
    3. There are no established association with phenotypes of serious mental disorders.

4. There are no legitimate concerns regarding under recognition of dual disability.
5. We should not accept our limitations of knowledge of psychopathology in validating psychopathology objectively when cognitions and communication may be impaired.

Answer: 1

PSYCHIATRIC ASSESSMENT

1. When people with learning disability are being assessed by psychiatrist

    1. It could be for emotional, behavioral, interpersonal, or family problems
    2. Allways presents with psychiatric disorders
    3. May not benefit from psychiatric input
    4. Psychiatric care is most effectively delivered by a multidisciplinary team approach
    5. 1 and 4

    Answer: 5

    Correct answers

    - It could be for emotional, behavioral, interpersonal, or family problems.
    - May not benefit from psychiatric input
    - Psychiatric care is most effectively delivered by a multidisciplinary team approach

    Wrong Answers

    - Allways presents with psychiatric disorders

2. In assessment of mental disorder in people with learning disability

    1. DSM-IV or the ICD-10 cannot be used as they are evidence based systems of classification relevant to all people

2. Reliability and validity of ICD-10, when applied to children with mental retardation is not established
3. Restrictions on dual diagnosis which are mutually exclusive (schizophrenia and Asperger's syndrome in DSM IV) are evidence based
4. Diagnostic Criteria for Psychiatric Disorders for use in adults with Learning Disabilities—DC-LD [77] is complementary to ICD-10
5. All the above

Answer: 4

Correct answers

- Diagnostic Criteria for Psychiatric Disorders for use in adults with Learning Disabilities-
- DC-LD [77] is complementary to ICD-10
- Restrictions on dual diagnosis which are mutually exclusive (schizophrenia and
- Asperger's syndrome in DSM IV) are increasingly being questioned

Wrong Answers

- DSM-IV or the ICD-10 cannot be used as they are evidence based systems of classification relevant to all people
- Reliability and validity of ICD-10 criteria when applied to children with mental retardation is not established
- Restrictions on dual diagnosis which are mutually exclusive (schizophrenia and
- Asperger's syndrome in DSM IV) are evidence based

3. Diagnostic Criteria for Psychiatric Disorders for use in adults with Learning. Disabilities-DC-LD

   1. Is a substitute for ICD-10
   2. Is a substitute for DSM IV
   3. Based on the principle of broadening the diagnostic categories to avoid diagnostic confusion

4. It is suitable for use by professionals untrained in making psychiatric diagnosis
   5. All the above

Answer: 3

Correct answers

- Based on the principle of broadening the diagnostic categories to avoid diagnostic confusion
- Complements current diagnostic systems

Wrong Answers

- Replaces ICD-10
- It is suitable for use by professionals untrained in making psychiatric diagnosis

4. In DSM IV

   1. Stereotypic movement disorder is not specific for people with learning disability
   2. Patterns of emotional and behavioural disturbance may occur exclusively in persons with mental retardation
   3. Specificity of symptoms face the same hurdles and criticisms of culture bound syndromes.
   4. Specificity of symptoms do not represent developmental level influencing the presentation of symptoms
   5. Specificity of symptoms do not represent intellectual ability influencing the presentation of symptoms

Answer: 3

Correct answers

- Stereotypic movement disorder is specific for people with learning disability

- Specificity of symptoms face the same hurdles and criticisms of culture bound syndromes.

Wrong Answers

- Stereotypic movement disorder is not specific for people with learning disability
- Patterns of emotional and behavioural disturbance may occur exclusively in persons with mental retardation
- Specificity of symptoms do not represent developmental level influencing the presentation of symptoms
- Specificity of symptoms do not represent intellectual ability influencing the presentation of symptoms

Specificity of symptoms may represent a marker of developmental level (Sexualised behaviour in puberty) and intellectual ability influencing the presentation of symptoms

5. Some generalizations about symptoms in people with learning disability having mental illness are relevant

   1. Symptoms are not just representing a decompensation or variable presentation due to cognitive and intellectual abilities.
   2. Adult patients with mild mental retardation are more likely to have externalizing symptoms
   3. If the people with mental retardation have psychotic symptoms, they are more likely to experience hallucinations without delusions
   4. All the above mentioned findings are similar to psycho-pathology in children in general
   5. Symptoms may represent developmental aspects of behaviour rather than being specific for the psychiatric disorder
   6. All the above

Answer: 6

6. With regard to specific psychiatric disorders in learning disability

   1. Conduct problems are more common
   2. Withdrawal is more common
   3. Attention and impulse control problems are more common
   4. 1, 2 and 3
   5. None of the above

   Answer: 4

   Correct answers

   - Conduct problems are more common
   - Withdrawal is more common
   - Attention and impulse control problems are more common

   Wrong Answers

   - Aggression is uncommon
   - Conduct disorder is more common

7. Population studies of children with learning disability show

   1. Autism and withdrawn behaviours are less common in those with severe learning disability
   2. Anxiety and aggressive behaviours are more common in those with milder levels of learning disability
   3. Autism and withdrawn behaviours are more common in those with severe learning disability
   4. Anxiety and aggressive behaviours are less common in those with milder levels of learning disability
   5. 2 and 3

   Answer: 5

   With regard to Standardized questionnaires for mental illness in learning disability

1. Psychiatric Assessment Schedule for Adults with Developmental Disability (PASADD) checklist is a screening instrument
2. PAS—ADD consists of a checklist of life events and symptoms, scored on a fourpoint scale.
3. Diagnostic Assessment for the Severely Handicapped II is a scale that is linked to DSM-IV. The anxiety, autism and schizophrenia subscales have been validated
4. The Cambridge Cognitive Examination is a group of tests that are included in the Cambridge Examination for Mental Disorders of the Elderly
5. Direct neuropsychological tests such as the Mini Mental State Examination are difficult to use reliably in adults with Down's syndrome
6. Matson Evaluation of Social Skills is a validated instrument to measure social skills among those with severe and profound mental retardation in individuals with Severe Retardation
7. The Minnesota Multiphasic Personality Inventory-168 (L) is a abbreviated version of the Minnesota Multiphasic Personality Inventory. It has substantial validity and testretest reliability in assessing adults and adolescent persons with mild and moderate learning disability
8. Developmental Behaviour Checklist is specific for use in children and adolescents with learning disability

---

8. Factor analysis of people with learning disability have identified the following relatively consistent groupings of disturbance

    1. Aggression or antisocial behaviour
    2. Social familiarity
    3. Non stereotypic behaviours
    4. Hypoactive behaviour
    5. Non repetitive communication problems

Answer: 1

Correct answers

- Aggression or antisocial behaviour
- Social withdrawal
- Stereotypic behaviours
- Hyperactive and disruptive behaviour
- Repetitive communication problems
- Anxiety fearfulness

Wrong Answers

- Social familiarity
- Non stereotypic behaviours
- Hypoactive behavior
- Non repetitive communication problems

9. With regard to mental retardation

   1. ICD 10 and DSM IV do not have a multiaxial classification
   2. Axis 2 on DSM IV multiaxial system is used to represent only mental retardation
   3. Axis 2 on DSM IV multiaxial system is used to represent only personality disorders
   4. Axis 2 on DSM IV multiaxial system is used to represent both mental retardation and personally disorders
   5. None of the above

Answer: 4

Correct answers

- ICD 10 and DSM IV have a multiaxial classification
- Axis 2 on DSM IV multiaxial system is used to represent both mental retardation and personally disorders

Wrong Answers

- ICD 10 and DSM IV do not have a multiaxial classification

10. In identifying psychiatric disorders

    1. Most DSM-IV diagnoses do not require patients describing their internal state
    2. Asking a person with severe mental retardation about hallucinations, delusions, or guilt is often productive.
    3. A clear onset of behavior problems may have diagnostic significance.
    4. None of the above
    5. All of the above

Answer: 3

Correct answers

- Most DSM-IV diagnoses require patients describing their internal state

Wrong Answers

- Asking a person with severe mental retardation about hallucinations, delusions, or guilt is often productive

11. Aspects of mental retardation that may influence diagnosis include

    1. Intellectual distortion
    2. Psychosocial masking
    3. Cognitive disintegration
    4. Baseline exaggeration
    5. All of the above

Answer: 5

Intellectual distortion refers to emotional symptoms that are difficult to elicit because of deficits in abstract thinking, communication and in receptive and expressive language skills.

Psychosocial masking is a term to represent limited social experiences influencing the content of psychiatric symptoms (e.g. mania presenting as a belief that one can drive a motorbike).

Cognitive disintegration is the decreased ability to tolerate stress, leading to anxiety or frustration induced decompensation.

Baseline exaggeration refers to increase in severity or frequency of a long term established maladaptive behavior after onset of psychiatric illness.

---

12. In diagnoses for mania and depression in mild learning disability

    1. Biologic signs can be useful in making diagnosis
    2. Comprehensive cognitive assessment is unnecessary to interpret behaviour in a developmental context
    3. Biological signs are not useful in making diagnosis
    4. Non specific symptoms without clear onset is characteristic
    5. Mood assessment may not be reliable

    Answer: 1

    Correct answers

    - Biologic signs can be useful in making diagnosis

    Wrong Answers

    - Non specific symptoms without clear onset is characteristic

13. Symptoms of psychopathology and emotions in learning disability

    1. May be indirectly expressed through developmental manifestation of behaviour similar to that seen in normal younger children
    2. The most frequent symptom is depression manifesting as irritable behaviour 56 MCQs

3. If expression of emotional and behavioural problem interpretation is impossible they cannot be classified under unclassified or organic brain syndromes
4. 1 and 2
5. None of the above

Answer: 4

Correct answers

- May be indirectly expressed through developmental manifestation of behaviour similar to that seen in normal younger children
- The most frequent symptom is depression manifesting as irritable behaviour

Wrong Answers

- If expression of emotional and behavioural problem interpretation is impossible they cannot be classified under unclassified or organic brain syndromes

14. With regard to cognitive abilities in autism

   1. Vary individually
   2. Can be generalised as being relatively better on performance tasks
   3. Can be generalised as being relatively worse on tasks that involve visual motor skills
   4. Can be generalized as performing relatively poor on verbal and social comprehension tasks 1 and 2
   5. 1, 2 and 3

Answer: 5

15. Childhood temperamental characteristics contribute to psychiatric disorders in learning disability

   1. Not useful predictors of psychiatric disturbance in children

2. Have no predictive validity in children
3. They are more relevant in mild mental retardation compared to more severe retardation.
4. There is no evidence regarding its relevance in later adulthood
5. Temperament may not be directly amenable to change, but may improve parental understanding and management skills.

Answer: 5

Correct answers

- Important predictors of psychiatric disturbance in children
- Temperament may not be directly amenable to change, but may improve parental understanding and management skills. It leads to better adaptation and the reduction in emotional and behavioural problems

Wrong Answers

- They are more relevant in mild mental retardation compared to more severe retardation
- There is no evidence regarding its relevance in later adulthood

16. Role of routine screening medical assessment in the psychiatric assessment of people with mental retardation.

1. It does not help to establish the cause of the mental retardation
2. It does not indicate presence of any associated medical condition
3. Young people with mental retardation have a lesser risk of medical problems
4. Young people with mental retardation have equal risk of medical problems
5. Young people with mental retardation have a higher risk of medical problems compared to general population

Answer: 5

17. Medical complications may be associated with known causes of learning disability

    1. Cardiac and bowel problems are not recognised in Down's syndrome
    2. Epilepsy is the not the most common neurological comorbidity associated with mental retardation
    3. Children with epilepsy have a equal risk of learning disability compared to general population
    4. Children with epilepsy have lesser risk of learning disability compared to general population
    5. Rates of psychopathology in people with mental retardation who have epilepsy are not increased except perhaps in those with poor seizure control

    Answer: 5

    Correct answers

    - Cardiac and bowel problems are recognized in Down's syndrome
    - Epilepsy is the not the most common neurological comorbidity associated with mental retardation

    Wrong Answers

    - Children with epilepsy have a equal or lesser risk of learning disability compared to general population

18. Children with learning disability when compared to other children in the community are

    1. Less likely to experience adverse experiences in life
    2. Less likely to undergo potential traumatic experiences like respite and institutional care
    3. Vulnerable group susceptible to social rejection
    4. They are less likely to be abused
    5. All of the above

Answer: 3

Correct answers

- Vulnerable group susceptible to social rejection
- Less likely to experience adverse experiences in life
- Less likely to undergo potential traumatic experiences like respite and institutional care

19. Cognitive abilities in learning disability

    1. Limit adaptability
    2. Limit understanding
    3. Limit coping abilities in socially stressful experiences
    4. May contribute to behavioural disturbance
    5. May be protective
    6. All of the above

    Answer: 6

20. The potential parental experiences of emotions of having a child with learning disability does not involve

    1. Over involvement,
    2. Grief
    3. Guilt
    4. Hostility
    5. Ambivalence
    6. Rejection
    7. Happiness
    8. None of the above

    Answer: 8

21. The following factors do not affect attachment in a child with learning disability

    1. The financial burden of care, parental emotions and relationships

2. Behavioural problems
3. Perceptual and sensory deficits
4. Communication difficulties
5. Normal Appetite

Answer: 5

22. Impaired attachment and parent-child interaction can be seen most commonly in

1. Learning disability
2. Normal child
   Learning Disability: MCQs 59
3. ADHD
4. Child with Autism
5. All of the above

Answer: 4

Correct answers

- Child with Autism

23. Impairment of the normal development is not worsened by

1. Neglect
2. Lack of stimulation
3. Lack of opportunity for play and social interaction
4. Over learning some motor sequences to master activities of daily living
5. Sensory impairment

Answer: 4

Correct answers

- Over learning some motor sequences to
- Mastering activities of daily living

Wrong Answers

- Neglect
- Lack of stimulation

24. With regard to parental stress in a family with a child having learning disability

   1. Correctable impairments screened early and rectified increases parental stress
   2. Having inappropriate help makes parents cope with the child better
   3. Mothers may not experience higher levels of stress than fathers.
   4. Increased maternal stress could be related to more maternal involvement and responsibility for care
   5. Is never culturally determined.

   Answer: 4

PSYCHIATRIC DIAGNOSIS

1. The components of a psychiatric assessment include

    1. Assessment of developmental aspects
    2. Assessment of communicative abilities
    3. Ideally performed in a multidisciplinary setting
    4. Should involve carers
    5. All the above

    Answer: 5

2. A detailed history can be obtained from

    1. The patient
    2. Other informants
    3. Parents Medical records
    4. None of the above
    5. 1 and 2

    Answer: 5

3. Guidelines useful for interviewing the person with mental retardation include

    1. It may not help by talking in a more concrete fashion,
    2. It helps to focus on the here and now
    3. Use words inappropriate to the person's level of understanding
    4. Leading questions are to be encouraged

5. Physical expressions and gestures to communicate with the person are unhelpful
   6. Storytelling may not facilitate communication
   7. 1, 2 and 4

   Answer: 2

   Correct answers

   - Talking to the person helps even if it appears that he/she might not understand
   - A person's receptive language skills are likely to exceed his or her expressive skills
   - It helps to focus on the here and now Leading questions are to be encouraged
   - Physical expressions and gestures to communicate with the person are unhelpful
   ---

4. Mood can be assessed in a non communicative patient by

   1. Observation of nonverbal interactions
   2. Psychomotor activity
   3. Eye contact
   4. Informants
   5. All the above

   Answer: 5

5. With regard to assessing aetiology of mental illness in people with learning disability

   1. Recent changes in the person's physical or social environment may not be relevant
   2. Loss of a favorite staff member is generally irrelevant
   3. Anniversary dates of losses and bereavement are not precipitants

4. Circumstantial patterns such as symptoms associated with a particular setting or time do not help to differentiate psychiatric disorder from a situational response.
5. A longitudinal history to correlate with concurrent events may point to aetiology

Answer: 5

6. Drug interactions can

   1. Worsen physical health
   2. Often precipitate aggression
   3. Can lead to self-injurious behavior
   4. All of the above
   5. None of the above

   Answer: 4

7. In management of psychiatric problems associated with mental illness

   1. Targetting primary psychiatric disorder is very effective
   2. Pharmacological treatments can worsen behaviour
   3. Pharmacological treatments may worsen behaviour
   4. Targeting symptoms is helpful if primary problem cannot be treated
   5. Establishing baseline rates of the target behavior to monitor response to treatment is unnecessary.

   Answer: 3

8. Abnormal involuntary movements

   1. Can be self injurious
   2. Are always self injurious
   3. Can occur only when the person is conscious
   4. Can occur only when the person is unconscious
   5. None of the above
   62 MCQs

Answer: 5

9. With regard to medication use in learning disability the following are not true

    1. Benzodiazepines with long half-lives may accumulate, leading to drowsiness and mental clouding
    2. Short-acting benzodiazepines may cause interdose rebound symptoms and worsening of anxiety just prior to scheduled doses
    3. Anticonvulsants may produce excessive sedation
    4. Antipsychotic drugs can have serious side effects, such as parkinsonism and akathisia that may be confused with worsening agitation
    5. Learning disability is not a vulnerability factor for drug induced

    Answer: 5

10. As part of the multidisciplinary team approach the evaluation

    1. Should be restricted to concerned learning disability team
    2. Should be restricted to concerned child psychiatry
    3. May be broadened to include, as needed, consultations other disciplines
    4. All the above
    5. None of the above

    Answer: 3

PSYCHIATRIC SYNDROMES

1. A number of identified genetic syndromes have

   1. Characteristic patterns of behaviour
   2. No characteristic patterns of behaviour
   3. An increased risk of specific psychiatric disorders
   4. 1 and 2
   5. All the above

   Answer: 4

2. In Down's syndrome

   1. No evidence of high prevalence of psychiatric disorders and behavioural problems
   2. Children with Down's syndrome are less likely to present with externalizing disorders
   3. Pattern changes in adolescence and young adulthood they are less likely to suffer from affective disorders and dementia
   4. A wide range of psychiatric disorders have been reported in this population
   5. None of the above

   Answer: 4

3. In people with Fragile X syndrome

   1. The most common genetic cause of mental retardation

2. Uniquely a differentiation in behavioural phenotypes has been described based on sex.
3. Boys are observed to be anxious, shy and avoiding eye contact.
4. Boys do not have problems with attention and hyperactivity
5. 1, 2 and 3

Answer: 10

Correct answers

- It is associated with characteristic behavioural problems
- Boys may sometimes present with stereotypy such as hand-flapping
- In Girls the symptoms are not usually as pronounced as that seen in boys
- There is no evidence suggesting an association with autism.
- Behavioural signs are non specific for diagnosis on their own

Wrong Answers

- Boys do not have problems with attention and hyperactivity

4. Children with Prader-Willi syndrome have

1. Severe mental retardation
2. Decreased appetite
3. Obsessive thoughts about food and a preoccupation with seeking food
4. They never need continuous supervision and a control over their eating habits in order to prevent life-threatening obesity
5. Obesity is uncommon

Answer: 3

5. In adults with Prader Willi syndrome

1. Symptoms are similar to childhood

2. Anxiety and low mood being more prevalent in older adolescents and adults
3. Maternal disomy of chromosome 15 is relatively more common
4. Deletion on the long arm of the paternal chromosome 15 is less common
5. None of the above

Answer: 2.

6. Smith Mageni's syndrome

    1. Chromosomal deletions at 17p11.2.
    2. Moderate mental retardation
    3. Behavioural phenotypes are characteristically hyperactive and aggressive
    4. They may have an unusual minimal need for sleep
    5. Prone to motor mannerisms such as 'self—hugging' when happy or excited
    6. All of the above

Answer: 6

7. Patau's syndrome is associated with

    1. Microcephaly
    2. Presence of corpus callosum
    3. cleft lip/ palate
    4. polydactyly
    5. 1, 3 and 4

Answer: 5

8. Edward's syndrome is associated with

    1. Flaccid baby with flexed limbs
    2. High set malformed ears
    3. protruding chin
    4. rocker-bottom feet
    5. more common in males

Answer: 4

9. Down's syndrome

   1. Trisomy 21
   2. 5 % is not due to translocation
   3. incidence does not increase with maternal age
   4. Incidence increases with paternal age
   5. None of the above

   Answer: 1

10. Cri du chat syndrome

    1. Deletion on chromosome 17
    2. Flaccid muscles
    3. No episodes of spasticity
    4. characteristic cry
    5. Not compatible with adult life

    Answer: 4

11. Self injurious behaviour among children with mental retardation include

    1. Head banging
    2. Pushing objects into body orifices
    3. Pulling nails
    4. Biting
    5. All of the above

    Answer: 5

12. William's syndrome

    1. No microdeletion on chromosome 7
    2. No mental retardation
    3. Have a specific profile of cognitive abilities with visuospatial and visuomotor deficits

4. Paradoxically a skill at recognizing facial features is reported in some children
   5. 3 and 4

Answer: 5

Expressive language may be well developed in a small subgroup and they may present as chatterboxes. They speak in an adult manner due to the stereotypic use of phrases learnt from adult conversation. In adolescence they may present with anxiety, hyperactivity, short attention span, and poor concentration.

---

13. Rett's syndrome

    1. Affects only females and is characterized by hand-wringing movements, variably progressing neurological deterioration and mental retardation.
    2. Genetic mutation (MECP2) on the X chromosome (Xq28) in 95% meeting criteria for typical RS
    3. Genetic mutation (MECP2) on the X chromosome (Xq28) in 50% meeting criteria for atypical RS
    4. The defective gene is MECP2, or methylcytosine binding protein,
    5. MECP 2 is lethal in males, accounting for its exclusive female presentation
    6. All of the above

Answer: 6

14. Some of the features of Rett's syndrome are

    1. Because of unusual X inactivation patterns, females with MECP2 mutations will never be normal or have milder forms of the disease
    2. Some women with MECP 2 mutation may not be identified unless they transmit the mutation to a daughter who develops Rett's Syndrome
    3. It is now known that RS cannot occur in males with Klinefelter syndrome (XXY) or somatic mosaicism

4. The child with RS usually shows an early period of abnormal development untill 6-18 months of life.
5. The child then gains communication skills and purposeful use of the hands and slowing of the rate of head growth becomes apparent.
6. Stereotyped hand movements and gait disturbances are early symptoms

Answer: 2

15. Angelman Syndrome

    1. Is not a genetic disorder
    2. No mental retardation
    3. No motor impairments
    4. Have vocal speech
    5. Muscular hypertonia
    6. Partial deletion of chromosome 15q11-q13

    Answer: 6

16. Among adults with learning disability

    1. Adults with Down syndrome have increased risk of early onset of Alzheimer's disease
    2. Mentally retarded adults without Down syndrome do not have an increased risk of Alzheimer's disease
    3. The number of older adults with mental retardation is increasing, because life span is increasing.
    4. 1, 2 and 3
    5. None of the above

    Answer: 4

17. With regard to associated disabilities in adults with learning difficulties

    1. 25% of mentally retarded adults have no useful speech
    2. 10% lack basic comprehension skills

Learning Disability: MCQs 67
3. 50% of adults cannot care for themselves
4. 50% half have a physical disability
5. All the above

Answer: 5

18. In improving quality of life among people with learning disability

   1. Prompt detection and treatment of mental or medical conditions is unhelpful
   2. Improving the life expectancy is not important
   3. Quality of life of people with mental retardation is not important
   4. Carers quality of life is not important
   5. None of the above

Answer: 5

There is no evidence supporting link between epileptic events and bouts of problem behavior has been documented for people with developmental disabilities. Treatment recommendations for epilepsy are generalised from normal population and may not always be appropriate.

---

19. Adults with mental retardation

   1. Have the same types of psychiatric disorders as adults of normal intelligence
   2. Accurate diagnosis is often easy to make.
   3. Diagnostic overshadowing, may increase identification of psychiatric conditions
   4. 1, 2 and 3
   5. None of the above

Answer: 1

20. Psychopathology among people with learning disability with psychosis

    1. Extrapolated from studies of adults with mild mental retardation and psychosis
    2. Delusions and hallucinations are present but are usually elaborate and systematized
    3. Occasionally impulsive, aggressive, and unpredictable behaviours do not dominate the clinical picture
    4. Delusions or hallucinations may be seen as agitation, sleeplessness, or aggression
    5. 1 and 4

    Answer: 5

21. The differential diagnosis for psychosis in learning disability includes

    1. Medical problems such as chronic pain
    2. Catatonic features
    3. Bereavement
    4. Presence of chronic persistent negative symptoms after an acute episode may aid in diagnosis
    5. All of the above

    Answer: 5

22. In people with learning disability having schizophrenia

    1. Subtypes of schizophrenia can be easily differentiated
    2. Can be made easily without communication
    3. Chronic persistent negative symptoms after an acute episode may aid in diagnosis
    4. The male: female ratio seems to be unequal
    5. Age of onset is not similar to the general population

    Answer: 3

    Correct answers

    - Subtypes of schizophrenia cannot be easily differentiated

- Cannot be made easily without communication
- Chronic persistent negative symptoms after an acute episode may aid in diagnosis
- The male: female ratio seems to be equal Age of onset is similar to the general population

Wrong Answers

- There appears to be specific relationship with epilepsy or chromosomal abnormalities
- Paranoid syndromes are never associated with disorders of hearing and vision
- Acute psychosis in children with mental retardation is common.
- In adults acute psychosis may be precipitated by stressful life events and recovery is never complete

23. In people with learning disability

   1. Milder forms of depression are not difficult to diagnose
   2. Dysthymia is not a recognised diagnosis in this subgroup.
   3. Research supports associations between depression and cognitive variables
   4. The leading cognitive theories of depression such as the diathesis-stress models cannot be generalised to all subpopulations including mental retardation.
   5. Biological symptoms are important indicators

Answer: 5

Prevalence studies suggests that some factors such as severe or profound developmental delay, sensory or physical disability, and certain genetic disorders and syndromes are associated with increased risk of developing self-injurious behavior. Self-injurious behavior can emerge prior to 3 years of age and that some of the children continue to engage in stereotypy, self-injurious behavior or proto-self-injurious behavior after they turn 3 years of age.

Proto—self-injurious behavior was defined as topographically similar to common forms of self-injurious behavior, but these topographies did not produce tissue damage. A strategy for reducing the prevalence of SIB is to identify effective early intervention and prevention strategies for young children who are at high risk of developing SIB. Motor stereotypies emerge in infancy and persist for young children with developmental delay rather than children developing new stereotypies throughout early childhood.

24. Behavioral equivalents for depression in individuals with mental retardation include

    1. Self-injury
    2. Aggression
    3. Withdrawal
    4. All of the above
    5. None of the above

    Answer: 4

25. About depression in people with learning disability

    1. Correlation between behavioral equivalents and self-reported depression has been established
    2. For diagnosing depression DSM-IV and ICD-10 criteria do not rely heavily on self-reports
    3. Standard criteria may be more appropriate for individuals with mild or moderate learning disability compared to severe
    4. Informant report instruments correlate well with self-reports of depression
    5. none of the above

    Answer: 3

    Correct answers

    - Informants usually describe valid accounts of the behavioral symptoms of depression, but report poorly on internalizing symptoms

Wrong Answers

- A similar trend has not been observed in the general population, with parents having less awareness of their children's internalizing than externalizing symptoms

26. In people with learning disability experiencing a bipolar disorder

   1. Prevalence rates range from 0.9% to 4.8%
   2. Estimates vary due to the difficulties in diagnosing bipolar disorder
   3. No evidence suggesting an increased prevalence of bipolar disorder in mental retardation.
   4. Diagnosis of bipolar affective disorder may be difficult in more severe forms of mental retardation
   5. All of the above

Answer: 5

27. About anxiety disorders in learning disability

   1. Children do not have simple fears characteristic of younger children such as fear of loud noises, the dark, insects, and animals
   2. Phobias cannot present in adults with mental retardation
   3. Separation anxiety can begin in much older children with a developmental age less than 5 years
   4. Systematic desensitization approach with relaxation and modeling is unhelpful as part of the management plan
   5. None of the above

Answer: 3

Among eating disorders Anorexia and Bulimia nervosa are rare. Mental retardation is a predisposing factor for other eating disorders such as pica and rumination. The ingestion of nonnutritive substances is called pica. The regurgitation and rechewing of food is called rumination.

28. A recognised form of adjustment disorder is

1. Bereavement and physical illness.
2. Bereavement cannot be a long absence of a carer
3. Bereavement cannot be normal
4. Parents do not play an important role in management
5. All of the above

Answer: 1

Obsessive-compulsive symptoms are common in children with mental retardation and autism. Insight into obsessions has been controversial, especially in children and generally not required for diagnosis. A range of behaviours can be considered as obsessive compulsive symptoms. These may include stereotypies and self-injurious behaviours. These are more common in children with autism There is no evidence that stereotypies act to reduce anxiety and they do not usually respond to treatments for anxiety

---

PSYCHOPHARMACOLOGY

Psychopharmacology

Which group of patients most frequently receive polypharmacy?

1. Patients with a mild learning disability
2. Patients with a severe learning disability
3. Patients with affective disorders
4. Patients with a schizophrenic psychosis
5. Patients with premorbid personality disorders
6. All of the above
7. None

Answer : 6

All the people under those categories are at increased risk of multiple medications. However people with schizophrenia are most at risk followed by mood disorders.

Polypharmacy does not include

1. Skillful combination of medication
2. A single Herbal medications alone
3. The combination of herbal medications with medications.
4. Using single chemical in a medication administered
5. Combining 2 different medications for the same outcome

Answer: 4

The following side effects are not true

1. St. John's wort does not induce hepatic enzymes
2. Ginko Boloba does not affect platelet function
3. Kava is not hepatotoxic
4. Fluvoxamine increases melatonin levels
5. Carbamazepine increases melatonin levels

Answer: 5

In people with learning disability

1. Underprescribing is common
2. Over prescribing is common
3. both under and over prescribing are common
4. behavioural changes do not indicate response to medication
5. Polypharmacy does not contribute to underprescribing

Answer: 3

With regard to side effects

1. Polypharmacy increases risk
2. High doses increase risk
3. learning disability increases risk
4. Probability of underprescription and side effects increases with polypharmacy
5. All the above

Answer: 5

In people with learning disability the following is not true

1. Polypharmacy is always useful
2. Underprescribing should be practised
3. Start medications at low dose medications but try upto the normal therapeutic doses.
4. Never reach doses used by people without learning difficulties
5. They are not very sensitive to side effects

Answer: 3

Reasons for use of polypharmacy in people with learning disability include

1. Better than monotherapy
2. Lesser side effects
3. more compliance
4. Good inter-rater reliability about need for multiple treatments
5. None of the above

Answer: 5

Reasons for using polypharmacy in people with learning disability include these reasons except:

1. Managing side effects of initial medication when it cant be stopped
2. To enhance effect of partial response to initial medications
3. To manage side effects of medication
4. To treat comorbidity
5. Reduce risk of side effects

Answer: 5

In a person with learning disability and schizophrenia

1. Smoking reduces the effectiveness of his treatment
2. Smoking reduces the rate of metabolism of antipsychotics.
3. The average plasma concentration of clozapine is lesser in smokers compared to non-smokers
4. Smoking does not affect any other organs other than liver
5. Smoking improves quality of life

Answer: 3

There is good evidence for combining this drug for optimising clozapine treatment in treatment resistant Schizophrenia :

1. Aripiprazole.
2. Haloperidol.

3. Lamotrigine.
4. Risperidone.
5. Quetiapine
6. Sulpiride

Answer: 6

APPENDIX 1

Learning disabilities continue to be quite significant limiting factors to a significant number of people. There has been many changes in assessment and management associated with a global sociocultural change in expectations regarding people with Learning Disability. The aims of this book are to help understand the basic concept of Learning Disability and its etiological factors along with understanding various ways of interpreting intelligence and measures of its impairment.

Assessment methods and management strategies for associated mental health disorders are also considered in view of the high associated incidence. Learning Disability is identified clinically as a developmental disorder. Research in etiology of Learning Disability has identified biological, environmental and psychological factors capable of producing deficits in intellectual function.

The co-occurrence of psychiatric illness with Learning Disability has been well established, and people with Learning Disability are more likely to suffer from mental ill health. However this association is non specific in most cases.

These conditions are often underdiagnosed due to issues such as "diagnostic overshadowing", the tendency by which clinicians tend to overlook additional psychiatric diagnosis once a diagnosis of Learning Disability is made; or "masking" in which the clinical characteristics of a mental disorder are masked by a cognitive, language or speech deficit.

People with Learning Disability share many mental health needs with the general population. The concept of 'normalisation', individual rights and respect for the wishes of individuals with Learning Disability has complemented the deinstitutionalised community care, carer support and psychopharmacological advances in psychiatry.

However, due to a variety of reasons their care has to be specifically tailored to meet these needs.

Learning Disability can be found as far back in history as the therapeutic papyri of Thebes (Luxor), Egypt, around 1500 B.C. These documents clearly refer to disabilities of the mind and body due to brain damage.

However the status and care received by individuals with Learning Disability varied greatly depending on cultures and periods of history.

In 1689, John Locke published his famous work entitled 'An Essay Concerning Human Understanding' explaining his landmark theory that an individual was born without innate ideas and described mind as a 'tabula rasa', a blank slate. This profoundly influenced the understanding of care and training provided to individuals with Learning Disability and continues to do so to this day. He also was the first person to differentiate between Learning Disability and mental illness.

A physician Jean-Marc-Gaspard Itard [1] who was hired in 1800 by the Director of the National Institutes for Deaf-Mutes in France to work with a boy named Victor revolutionized the application of learning principles of the time in teaching Victor, a young boy, who had apparently lived his whole life in the woods of south central France. Based on the work of Locke emphasizing the importance of learning through the senses, he developed a broad educational program for Victor to develop his senses, intellect, and emotions. After 5 years of training, Victor continued to have significant difficulties in language and social interaction though he acquired more skills and knowledge than many of Itard's contemporaries believed possible at the time. Itard's humanistic educational approach became widely accepted and even to this day it is used in the education of the deaf.

Itard also supervised Edouard Seguin who developed a comprehensive approach to the education of children with Learning Disability. His approach began with sensory training including vision, hearing, taste, smell, and eye-hand coordination. In 1850, Seguin was lured to the

United States and became a driving force in the education of individuals with Learning Disability. In 1876, he founded what would become the American Association on Metal Retardation. Many of Seguin's techniques are still in use today.

Alfred Binet developed an intelligence scale that was translated by Henry Goddard to English. Edgar Doll developed the Vineland Social Maturity Scale to assess the daily living skills and adaptive behavior of individuals suspected of having Learning Disability. Psychologists and educators now stepped in with medical professionals in believing that it was possible to determine and measure who had Learning Disability and how to quantify it and provide them with appropriate education.

These institutions were initially more educational in nature but became custodial centres breeding institutionalism. The United States passed the Education for the Handicapped Act in 1975, which guaranteed the appropriate education of all children with Learning Disability and developmental disabilities, from school age through 21 years of age.

The implications indirectly extend to include management of mental illness coexisting with Learning Disability.

The terminology used for this group of individuals has varied with time. In North America the broad term 'developmental delay' is preferred by many parents and caregivers. The term developmental disability, physical or psychiatric delay, delayed puberty, Intellectual disability and learning disability are increasingly being used as a synonym for people with significantly below-average intelligence. Mental handicap is the term used by the UK Mental Health Act 1983. However the American Association on Learning Disability continues to use the term Learning Disability which is adopted by the Diagnostic and Statistical Manual IV-DSM

Due to concern about the over identification or misidentification of Learning Disability, particularly in minority populations, the definition was revised in 1973. A 1977 revision modified the upper Intelligence Quotient (IQ) limit to 70-75 to account for measurement error. IQ performances resulting in scores of 71 through 75 were only consistent with Learning Disability when significant deficits in adaptive behavior were present.

Association of mental illness with Learning Disability has developed significantly recently. Kraepelin described 'Pfropfschizophrenie' i.e. schizophrenia in people with Learning Disability [10]. He also differentiated it from "oligophrenia", which is associated with low psychic or mental functioning without psychopathology in people with mild retardation.

In general, the psychopathology suffered by patients with Learning Disability resemble those of normal individuals. However, they occur at a greater-than-normal incidence.

A diagnosis of Learning Disability by itself does not amount to a disorder. Many children and adults with Learning Disability live in the community with very little need of involvement from health and social services.

The American Association of Learning Disability decided by consensus in 1993 that the term Mental retardation' was most appropriate term and is defined as 'a disability characterized by significant limitations both in intellectual functioning and in adaptive behavior as expressed in conceptual, social, and practical adaptive skills. This disability originates before the age of 18 years'. It is used internationally.

Five assumptions are essential to the application of the definition. These are

(1) Limitations in present functioning within the context of community, age, peers and culture.
(2) Valid assessment should include cultural and linguistic diversity as well as differences in communication, sensory, motor, and behavioral factors.
(3) Within an individual, limitations often coexist with strengths and these need to be evaluated systematically.
(4) An important purpose of assessment and describing limitations is to develop a profile of needed supports.
(5) With appropriate personalized supports over a sustained period, the life and quality of functioning of the person with Learning Disability generally will improve.

The International statistical classifications of diseases and related health problems, 10th edition—ICD 10 [15] and DSM IV [7] refer to substantial limitations in present functioning characterised by significant sub-average intellectual functioning existing concurrently with related impaired limitations in two or more of the following applicable skills areas: communication, healthcare, home living, social skills, community use, self direction, health and safety, functional, academic leisure and work and manifest before the age of 18.

These definitions regard Learning Disability as a state rather than as a stable trait Psychopathology in Learning Disability may vary depending on the cognitive and intellectual ability and also on the level of communication. In addition neurological and genetic phenotypes of Learning Disability may present with unique symptoms.

Psychopathology associated with Learning Disability can be discussed in 3 ways:

(1) Developmental psychology of Learning Disability
(2) psychopathology of co morbid physical disorders
(3) psychopathology of co morbid psychiatric disorders

There are common and unique characters in psychopathology of co morbid psychiatric disorders in people with Learning Disability.

1. Psychology and descriptive psychopathology of Learning Disability

- People with Learning Disability have difficulty in acquisition of basic living, educational, and social skills that is apparent early in life together with evidence of a significant intellectual impairment.
- They may have sensory impairments and very substantial care needs.
- In a significant proportion with subtle signs of early developmental delay, together with evidence of learning difficulties only become apparent at school.
- Assessment is essentially to determine need and to inform the types of intervention and treatments, whether educational, medical, psychological, or social, that are likely to be effective.
- Intelligence is not a unitary characteristic but is assessed on the basis of a large number of different more or less specific skills
- The general tendency is for skills to develop relatively to similar levels in each person but there can be large discrepancies.

- Some people with Learning Disability can have severe impairments in one particular area, or may have a particular area of higher skill.
- Adaptive functioning has to be measured against what would be expected for a person of that age, and socio cultural background.
- Challenging behaviour is a commonly used term to describe unexplained behavioural disturbance in people with Learning Disability.
- The best way to deal with challenging behaviour is to find out the cause of the behaviour. This may necessitate observation by carers for a behavioural analysis. Sometimes a person with challenging behaviour may need medication if psychosocial interventions do not produce significant change.

2. Psychopathology of co morbid conditions of neurological and genetic origin

   - There are many identified genetic disorders associated with Learning Disability.
   - Many of these disorders play a causal role in Learning Disability. However, most of the causal relationships must be inferred by epidemiological studies.
   - The American Association on Learning Disability subdivides the disorders that may be associated with Learning Disability into three: prenatal causes, perinatal causes, and postnatal causes.
   - Learning Disability is both a symptom of other disorders as well as a unique syndrome or disorder.
   - The most common factor associated with severe Learning Disability has been chromosomal abnormality, particularly Down's syndrome
   - neurological conditions associated with Learning Disability include epilepsy and various other neurological syndromes. Their relevance is never to be ignored and a need for a detailed neurological assessment is important.
   - They are also relevant in management since the medications used to treat them can interact and sometimes present with psychiatric side effects.

3. Psychopathology of co morbid psychiatric disorders/mental illness

   - Developmental and intellectual abilities may restrict expression of psychopathology

- Clarity and structure of thought and perceptual abnormalities like delusions and hallucinations may be restricted
- There are no universally agreed criteria for diagnosis d) Often diagnosis is based on behavioural observations and course of illness due to limitations in communication

Estimating prevalence of mental disorders in people with Learning Disability id difficult. Epilepsy, mental illness, obesity, and general unfitness are especially common in this population.

International differences in prevalence, quality of life, morbidity, and life expectancy for people with Learning Disability arevery significant and cannot be explained easily.

Within the same population prevalence varies between similar births cohorts (concurrent age groups). Greater variation is expected in developing countries, especially where there are environmental factors like iodine deficiency disease. Down syndrome is often the largest aetiological group.

It is vitally important to identify locally preventable etiological factors and strategically manage them. Prevalence of psychiatric disorders in people with Learning Disability is restricted by all the drawbacks of epidemiological identification of Learning Disability.

Study of aetiological factors among people with Learning Disability has provided insights into the multifactorial causative factors contributing to the aetiology of mental illness. The historical emphasis on biological causative factors including genetics has yielded good results in finding the aetiology of Learning Disability.

Though the results of association between Down's syndrome and psychiatric disorders remains unclear, the debate has improved the understanding and demystifying aetiology of challenging behaviour in people with Learning Disability. There is increasing evidence that such behavioural disturbances are not always related to psychiatric disorders. A sequence of psychosocial and environmental events can cause these symptoms. This emphasises psychosocial and environmental factors as important therapeutically modifiable factors. Such interventions have proven long term benefits and form an important component of management.

The various ways in which psychiatric disorders could be comorbid with learning disability could be discussed as follows,

> Chance association of psychiatric disorder with Learning Disability
> Increased incidence of psychiatric disorders among people with Learning Disability
> Decreased incidence of psychiatric disorders among people with Learning Disability

The problems in evaluating such probable associations have presented some unique challenges such as

> Diagnostic overshadowing—intellectual disability and communication difficulties obscure the diagnosis of a mental health disorder
> Importance of neurodevelopmental processes in abnormal behavior, coping and resilience.
> Lack of specificity of aetiological association to Learning Disability and psychiatric disorders
> Presence of co morbid neurodevelopment disorders
> Lack of evidence for later/earlier onset of psychiatric illnesses
> Lack of evidence specifically studying association between Learning Disability and psychiatric disorders

APPENDIX 2

Important Concepts in Learning disability	
Advocated treatment without mechanical restraints	Conolly (1794-1866)
Anxiety	Lewis
Crisis Intervention	Linderman (1944), Caplan (1961)
Gestalt Therapy	F. Perls
Hypnotherapy	Milton Erikson
Illness Behaviour	Mechanic
Interpersonal therapy	Sullivan
Malarial treatment of neurosyphilis	Wagner von Jauregg
breaking of the chains of the inmates of the Saltpetriere	Pinel (1745-1826)
Social Learning	Albert Bandura
The Sick Role	Parsons
Therapeutic Community	Maxwell Jones
Token Economies	Ayllon & Azrin
Transactional analysis	F. Berne

Hypnotism	James Braid
The Four A's of Schizophrenia	Eugene Bleuler
"Bell and Pad" treatment of enuresis	Mowrer & Mowrer
Autism	Leo Kanner
Dissociation	Janet
ECT	Cerletti and Bini
Psycholinguistics	Naom Chomsky
Cognitive Dissonance	Leon Festinger
First Rank Symptoms of Schizophrenia	Kurt Schneider
Aversion Therapy, Covert Sensitization	Rachman & Teasdale
Exposure Therapy	Marks, Gelder, and Mathews
Cognitive Theory of Depression	Aaron Beck
Learned Helplessness	Seligman & Maier
systematic densensitization	Joseph Wolpe

APPENDIX 3

Intelligence

Intelligence is a complex set of characteristics including possessing of knowledge, the ability to efficiently use knowledge to reason adaptively in different settings.

In 1904 the French Government employed Alfred Binet to look into special educational programs for children failing in school and he was a pioneer in developing measures of intelligence. In 1916, Lewis Terman at Stanford University developed an English version, the Stanford-Binet Test. The measure Intelligence Quotient was defined as:

$$\frac{\textit{Mental age} \times 100}{\text{Chronological age}}$$

1. The average score obtained by people at each age level is assigned the IQ value of 100 and it reflects your *relative* standing within a population of your age
2. IQ tests given before the age of 7 do not correlate very highly with scores on IQ tests given later because test items used for young children are different and cognitive abilities change rapidly in the early years
3. IQ tests now include more than one scale, so that areas most influenced by culture, such as vocabulary, can be assessed separately
4. there are some sex differences among boys and girls

Boys	Girls
better at skills involving spatial relations have a greater range of IQ more gifted in specific tasks	have better linguistic ability, but not necessarily vocabulary have higher IQ scores in childhood

boys:
- are better at skills involving spatial relations
- have a greater range of IQ
- are more gifted

girls:
- have better linguistic ability, but not necessarily vocabulary
- have higher IQ scores in childhood

APPENDIX 4

Intelligence Tests

The Wechsler Adult Intelligence Scale (WAIS)
6 **verbal** subtests
- general information
- comprehension
- vocabulary
- arithmetic
- digit span
- similarities

5 **performance** subtests
- block design
- object assembly
- picture completion
- digit symbol
- picture arrangements

* the WAIS allows computation of a *verbal IQ*, a *performance IQ*, and an *overall IQ*

(Ravens) Progressive Matrices
- measures non-verbal IQ
- consists of a diagram-completion test which exists in three versions:
    - Standard, for average ability
    - Coloured, for children and those of lower ability
    - Advanced, for those of above average ability

Organic Brain Dysfunction

Bender-Gestalt Test
- can be used in the assessment of:
    - mental retardation
    - aphasias
    - psychoses
    - neuroses
    - malingering

APPENDIX 5

Definitions

- *Impairment*—any loss or abnormality or psychological, physiological, or anatomical structure or function
- *Disability*—any reduction or lack (resulting from impairment) of ability to perform an activity in the manner or within the range considered normal for a human being
- *Handicap*—a disadvantage for the individual, resulting from impairment or disability that limits the fulfillment of a role that is normal for that individual. May be in dimensions of physical independence, mobility, occupation, social integration, economic self-sufficiency, orientation, or other

ICD-10
- *Mental Retardation (MR)*—a condition of arrested or incomplete development of the mind, which is especially characterized by impairment of skills manifested during the developmental period, which contribute to the overall level of intelligence, i.e. cognitive, language, motor, and social abilities

DSM-IV
1. Subaverage intellectual functioning, IQ < 70
2. Concurrent deficits in ≥ 2 skills areas:
   - communications
   - self-care
   - home living
   - social/ interpersonal skills
   - use of community resources

- self-direction
- academic skills
- leisure
- work
- health and safety

3. onset before age 18

Coding

	IQ range (ICD-10 and DSM-IV)
Mild MR	50-69
Moderate MR	35-49
Severe MR	20-34
Profound MR	<20

APPENDIX 6

Causes of Mental retardation

Infections (Can occur prenatally, at birth or postnatally)
- Congenital CMV
- Congenital Rubella
- Congenital Toxoplasmosis
- Encephalitis
- HIV infection
- Listeriosis
- Meningitis

Chromosomal abnormalities
- Chromosome deletions (like cri du chat syndrome)
- Chromosomal translocations (a gene located in an unusual spot on a chromosome, or located on a different chromosome than usual)
- Defects in the chromosome or chromosomal inheritance (such as fragile X syndrome, Angelman syndrome, Prader-Willi syndrome)
- Defects in chromosome numbers (such as Down syndrome)

Environmental
- Emotional Deprivation in early childhood

Genetic abnormalities and inherited metabolic disorders
- Adrenoleukodystrophy
- Galactosemia
- Hunter's syndrome

- Hurler's syndrome
- Lesch-Nyhan syndrome
- Phenylketonuria
- Rett's syndrome
- San-filippo syndrome
- Tay-Sachs disease
- Tuberous sclerosis

Metabolic
- Congenital hypothyroidism
- Hypoglycemia
- Reye's syndrome
- Hyperbilirubinemia and Kernicterus

Nutritional
- Malnutrition

Toxic
- Intrauterine exposure to alcohol, cocaine, amphetamines, and other drugs
- Lead poisoning
- Methylmercury poisoning

Trauma (before and after birth)
- Intracranial hemorrhage before or after birth
- Lack of oxygen to the brain before, during, or after birth
- Severe head injury

Unexplained (this largest category is for unexplained occurrences of mental retardation)

REFERENCES

American Association on Learning Disability. Learning Disability: Definition, Classification, and Systems of Supports. 10th Edition. Washington DC: American Association on Mental Retardation; 2002.

American Psychiatric Association. Diagnostic and Statistical Manual of Classification of diseases and related health problems. 4th edition. Washington DC: American Psychiatric Association; 1994.

Cooper, S. A. (1997). Epidemiology of psychiatric disorders in elderly compared with younger adults with learning disabilities. *British Journal of Psychiatry,* 170, 375-380.

Deb, S. (1997). Mental disorder in adults with Learning Disability and epilepsy. *Comprehensive Psychiatry,* 38(3), 179-184.

Deb, S. and Joyce, J. (1998). Psychiatric illness and behavioural problems in adults with learning disability and epilepsy. *Behavioural Neurology,* 11(3), 125-129.

Dobson, F. and Michael, A. Mental Health Act. UK: Department of Health; 1983.

Girimaji, S.R., Srinath, S. and Seshadri, S.P. (1994). A clinical study of infants presenting to a Learning Disability clinic. *Indian Journal of Pediatrics,* 61(4), 373-378.

Irish College of Psychiatrists (2004). Proposed model for the delivery of a mental health service to people with intellectual disability: Occasional Paper (OP58). *Psychiatric Bulletin,* 28, 345-346.

Jaffe, JH. "Learning Disability." In: Sadock, B.J. and Sadock, V.A (Eds), Comprehensive Textbook of Psychiatry, 7th edition, Philadelphia, PA: Lippincott Williams and Wilkins; 2000.

McLaren, J. and Bryson, S. E. (1987) Review of recent epidemiological studies in mental retardation: prevalence, associated disorders, and etiology. *American Journal of Mental Retardation,* 92, 243-254.

National Assembly for Wales. Welsh Health Survey 1998. Wales: *HMSO;* 1999. Patel, P., Goldberg, D. and Moss, S. (1993) Psychiatric morbidity in older people with moderate and severe learning disability—II: The prevalence study. *British Journal of Psychiatry,* 163, 481-491.

Qureshi, H. The Size of the Problem. In: Emerson E., McGill P. and Mansell J (Eds), *Severe Learning Disabilities and Challenging Behaviours,* Chapman and Hall; 1994.

Royal College of Psychiatrists. Diagnostic Criteria for Psychiatric Disorders for Use with Adults with Learning Disabilities (DC-LD): London: Royal College of Psychiatrists; 2001

Rutter, M; Tizard, J. and Witmore, K. Education, Health, and Behaviour. London: Longman; 1970

Rutter, M., Tizard, J., Yule, W., Graham, Y., and Whitmore, K. (1976). Isle of Wright studies 1964-1974. *Psychological Medicine,* 7, 313-332.

Sheerenberger, RC. A history of Learning Disability. Baltimore: Brookes Publishing Co; 1983.

Srinath, S. and Girimaji, S.C. (1999). Epidemiology of child and adolescent mental health problems and Learning Disability. *NIMHANS Journal,* 17, 355-366.

The Arc of the United States. Preventing Learning Disability: A Guide to the Causes of Learning Disability and Strategies for Prevention. Silver Spring, MD.2001. (http://www.thearc.org/publications/prevention.pdf).

World Health Organization. International Classification of Impairments, Disabilities and Handicaps. Geneva: WHO; 1980.

World Health Organization. International statistical classification of diseases and related health problems. 10th revision. Geneva: WHO; 1992.

Zenderland, L. Measuring minds: Henry Herbert Goddard and the origins of American intelligence testing. Cambridge: Cambridge University Press; 1998.

www.ingramcontent.com/pod-product-compliance
Lightning Source LLC
Chambersburg PA
CBHW021956170526
45157CB00003B/1020